The Lemon Bar Queen

The
LEMON BAR
QUEEN

A Memoir of Love,
Baking, and Memory Loss

JODI MELSNESS

ISBNs: 978-1-7331757-0-8 (paperback); 978-1-7331757-1-5 (kindle); 978-1-7331757-2-2 (ePub)

Library of Congress Control Number: 2019906825
Printed in the United States of America
First Printing: 2019
23 22 21 20 19   5 4 3 2 1

Book designed and set in type by Mayfly Design

"For Good" from the Broadway musical *Wicked*
Music and Lyrics by Stephen Schwartz
Copyright © 2003 Stephen Schwartz

Cold Lake Publishing
Plymouth, Minnesota

For inquiries or orders, contact Jodi at jodi.melsness@gmail.com
or visit thelemonbarqueen.com

For my parents, Russell and Jeanne Lundell.
With love, from your brown-eyed girl.

And for all families dealing with memory loss
and doing the very best they can, every single day.

Contents

Prelude

I'm listening to the quiet, gentle whir of my dad's oxygen concentrator as I sit cross-legged on the worn yellow carpet in our living room. I can just see my dad through the door. He is lying in his hospital bed in the den, and the sounds of golf are coming from the TV. My mom is busy in the kitchen wiping off counters. I can smell freshly brewed coffee. She will not sit down. I know she is trying to keep busy by baking and cleaning. I can tell she is a nervous wreck but doesn't want anyone to know.

In front of me is a stack of papers from Bremer Bank. My dad has given me the task of organizing their bank CDs in the order of maturity. I am overwhelmed and anxious about this project, but I don't want to let him know. I can feel this is of great importance to him.

One of the things I notice is that they have more money invested than I thought, and I am proud they were so organized. What I am surprised at is that he is trusting me to take care of all of Mom's needs.

My dad has advanced lung cancer. He stopped his chemo treatments two weeks ago and has declined quickly. I asked for a leave of absence from my nursing job in Minneapolis and drove the two hours to my hometown of Starbuck, Minnesota. It's the first time I have left my almost four-year-old and my husband for any length of time. I am reminded of all the good memories of my hometown.

As I look up from the papers, my dad motions for me to come into the den. Over the last few days, I have watched him slowly fade away. During this time, my mom has been bone-weary but refuses to give up on the thought that he will get better.

Today they have been married four days shy of sixty years—an eternity in our day and age.

I slowly get up from the floor and go into the den. My dad's oxygen cannula is half out of his nose. I gently put it back in. I look at the time and apply a new fentanyl pain patch to keep him comfortable. He is looking pale and thinner than I have ever seen him. He tells me he is thirsty, and I give him a drink of water and fix his rumpled sheets. I sit by the bed and he looks at me with a look of such sadness. "Jodi, Jodi, Jodi." He softly repeats my name over and over and continues to stare at me.

"Your mother is getting more confused every day," he says. "I know I have told you about her forgetting her purse at the café, and she is forgetting things in the oven. Last week, she forgot the eggs in the brownies. When I'm gone, it's up to you to take care of her. You must look after her. Whatever you need, I have spelled out all of it in those papers you have. Sell the house and do what you feel is best for her. I know you will take good care of her."

The whole time he is speaking, he is holding my hand and I can hear Mom on the phone giving someone an update on how he is doing. She is not a part of the conversation. I wish she was right here with me. She would realize that my dad wants me to take care of her and that she will be all right after he is gone.

"Dad, I've noticed she's been more repetitive on the phone and I can see some of the forgetfulness," I say. "Please don't worry about Mom. I will make sure I take care of her just like you did. Please don't worry."

I know he wants to say more but the medication is making

him drowsy. The cancer is taking my dad and leaving my mom without a husband and my brother and me without a father.

Before I go to bed, I give my dad a sponge bath and I feel the warm tears stream down my face. My brother's girlfriend, Heather, has come to help me because I don't want my mom to lift him. I know he will die soon. I can see it in his breathing. And he has stopped verbalizing. His death is coming.

He has lost fifteen pounds from his once-strong body and he can barely move himself without help. I see the scars that make him who he is. The scar on his back from falling out of a deer stand. The scar on his fingers from the surgery to separate his webbed fingers at birth and the reason he never wore a wedding band.

As I wash his face, I can see the big faded scar from his heart and lung surgeries, which he recovered from just in time to walk me down the aisle at our Lutheran church. He is full of the marks that make up his eighty-one years.

I finish putting lotion on his legs, and my mom comes in to ask if we are hungry. I'm not sure if she realizes that her husband will die soon. I try to keep her busy so she doesn't feel she needs to help turn him. I ask if she will make me something. She has always felt the need to be useful, and the kitchen is her sanctuary. She has barely sat down since I arrived, and I am worried about her.

When we both get ready for bed, I ask Mom if she wants to sleep beside Dad in the twin bed next to his hospital bed. I slept in that bed last night, although not much sleep happened. My nursing instincts kept me listening for any breathing or pain issues. I could also hear the concentrator all night long, humming along, keeping my dad comfortable. Little would I know that years later, after all the patients on oxygen I have taken care of, I can still picture that night before my dad died and hear the hum of that concentrator.

During the night there is a terrible thunderstorm, the kind that shakes the windows. Rain continues to fall in sheets against the windows, and I can feel the wind through the old windows in their house. Again I can't sleep. It's 2 a.m. and I am worried and scared. I'm in an unfamiliar bed and my parents' bedroom is lit up like the Fourth of July. When I was a child, my dad always told us that when it thundered loudly it meant God was bowling in heaven, and I believed that for the longest time. I told my girls the same thing. Even to this day, my younger daughter reminds me when it is storming outside that "Papa is bowling in heaven!"

I crawl out of their bed and find my way around the house using the lightning for illumination. Loud cracks of thunder continue. I turn the corner toward the den and I can hear the humming that I am supposed to hear, but I can't hear my dad's loud mouth breathing. I look at my mom and she is sound asleep, gently snoring on her side.

I walk over to my dad's side and I can tell that he is gone. He is a grayish color and his head is off to the side. He looks like he is taking a peaceful nap, the kind that he always tried to sneak in after a long day out in the farm fields. I reach for the oxygen tubing and pull it out of his nose. I close his eyes and mouth and sit with him for a moment before I wake up my mom. "I love you and will miss you, Dad."

I'm not sure how long he has been gone. When I went to bed at eleven, I told Mom to come and get me if she needed me. But I'm sure she fell asleep, exhaustion finally taking over. I wonder if it's really him causing all that racket from up above. Maybe it's not God, but really Dad bowling a perfect score. One last goodbye for the both of us.

I slowly wake up Mom. She's disoriented and confused. "Dad is gone, Mom," I tell her. She puts her hands on her face and cries. "Oh, Russell!" she moans. My nursing role kicks in and I call hospice, which in turn contacts the mortuary. I sit Mom down and tell her I will take care of everything. The hospice nurse must come out and pronounce him "dead." I told her she didn't really need to come since she knows I'm a nurse and it's something I've done many times. She tells me that it's their protocol. It takes her two hours to get to our home from Alexandria because of the storm.

I think of all the times I have prepped bodies of patients, making sure they are cleaned up before the mortuary comes. Cleaning, rolling, wiping fluids, combing hair, making sure the blanket and sheets are just so. It's the role of a nurse. You want them to look nice, even in death. I am ashamed to say I could not be in the same room with my dad. It was a very difficult moment knowing his body is there but he is not.

After everyone leaves, it is 4:30 a.m. I am exhausted, and I want to call my husband, Steve, but I wait until morning. I also need to call my brother. I am dreading telling him.

My mom has made some coffee and she brings it to me outside. I'm sitting on a long brown church pew that my parents inherited from somewhere, which is set up by their garden. I am watching the sun come up through the trees. The terrible storm is over, my dad has stopped bowling and I know that I have a lot to do today.

Mainly I sit and think about Mom. How will I do this from afar? What will she do without him? When should I get her to see a neurologist? Who is the best neurologist I know? Who will take care of her daily needs?

Yesterday, the day before he died, he made me promise to take care of her. I think about that promise as I'm watching the birds eat strawberries out of their garden. The birds are singing. I hear the phone start to ring. The day is about to begin, and I say a little prayer for all of us. But mainly for me.

PART ONE

The New Beginning, August 2007

I hardly gave my mom a chance to mourn. The day after my dad's funeral I told her friends that she would be staying with me for a few weeks and to keep an eye on her home. It was now just my mom in the home. I didn't want her to be alone.

On the car ride down to Minneapolis, I could see how tired she was from the weeks of stress. She talked a little, I talked too much, trying to take her mind off her husband's death. She slept most of the way.

I have travel plans for us, I tell her when she wakes up. We can go on road trips to all sorts of destinations. I name a few that I have been interested in: Galena, Illinois; Door County; Red Wing; Bayfield; and Madeline Island. All places that are close. I know how much she and my dad loved to travel.

We pull into the driveway and the one person who can make Mom smile is standing in the driveway, my soon-to-be four-year-old daughter, Sophia. No one makes my mom's heart melt more than she does. She loves to tell people how many years she waited for Sophia. Trust me, I have heard the story repeatedly. If you knew my mom, you would have heard the same story also.

My mom and dad were seventy-eight when Sophia was born and no one was more loved than she was when she arrived.

We settle Mom into her room in our basement and we order Chinese food. Mom looks noticeably thinner. I know she will finally eat a meal she likes. She always orders the same thing: chow mein. She eats half of it and saves the rest for the next day. She lived through the Depression and old habits are hard to break.

The next day we attend a golf tournament in honor of my cousin Tom, who took his own life in 2003 when I was pregnant with Sophia. He was special to my parents and he was also their godchild. We all grieved for Tom.

I know Mom will enjoy being around people, and her sister Gloria will be there, along with her nieces and nephews. Mom thrives on being social. At the banquet, everyone acknowledged her loss. On the car ride home she says she felt very loved. She starts to slowly cry at a stoplight and now we are both crying. "I miss Russell!" This will not be the last time we cry together. I miss him too. I begin to wonder how I'll be able to handle taking care of my own family and Mom.

The Surprise

A year after we had Sophia, my husband, Steve, and I found out that we were pregnant again. It was a surprise, but we were excited. We told both of my parents and Steve's mother that we were expecting. My mom could talk of nothing else. She telephoned all her friends. And, as a small town goes, each of the 1,200 people in Starbuck knew I was pregnant by the end of the day.

But, as life goes, I miscarried at thirteen weeks. I had fallen a few days before while taking the blood pressure of a retired physician with memory loss whom I adored. He had a school chair with wheels on it and I tipped right out of it. I was so embarrassed as he tried to get me up off the floor. I doubt that had anything to do with it, but it was difficult to call both sets of parents and tell them we were no longer pregnant.

A year after our miscarriage, we became pregnant again. Again, we were thrilled. Our first calls were to our parents. And again, I'm sure half of Starbuck knew I was pregnant again before I put the phone down. I was happy, yet cautious.

I was taking the garbage out to the end of the street on a snowy night and I fell on the slippery street. I didn't hurt myself and I hoped no one had seen me fall. I came in and told Steve what had happened, but I knew I was okay. The next day on my nursing visits I started to bleed and I knew that I was again losing our baby. It was again thirteen weeks. I just could not get past that awful week. I drove myself to the doctor's office and went through an awful exam. Steve wanted to be there, but there was no reason for him to come. I waited in that office for one full hour, only for them to tell me they didn't know what happened and that my fall most likely wasn't the reason for my loss. I know that logically as a nurse, but I still felt incredibly sad and empty. It was a difficult time for our little family of three.

I came home and took a bath. Sophia entered the bathroom, as any three-year-old does, and saw me crying in the tub. "Mommy, why are you sad?" Not wanting to tell her, I said I didn't feel good and the bath was helping me.

I got out of the tub and called my mom, who immediately started to cry. My dad grabbed the phone and shared with me that his own mother, Hazel, lost two babies in between him and his sister and to "get back on that horse!" as only my dad would say. I know for a fact that my mom had a hard time telling her friends the news because many of her friends asked how I was doing with my pregnancy, weeks after our loss. The loss for us was just as great for her.

It was around Christmas, three months after my dad died, that I found out I was pregnant again. Steve and I swore we were not going to tell anyone, and we didn't until I was halfway through my pregnancy. We finally told our family that we had made it to twenty weeks and my mom was happy, yet worried. I told her I was feeling fine and had not had any falls. We had a scan of the baby and it was a girl and everything looked normal.

July 13, 2008, eleven months after my dad died, Emme Marie Melsness entered the world. I remember the day that my mom, a grandma now for the second time, touched her sweet face. "I'm so proud of you!" she cried. Both of my girls are named after my mom and she loved that we kept the name Marie, which is her middle name, and my great-aunt's name, who also battled memory loss.

I've shared with a few of my friends that I felt Emme was really a parting gift that my dad gave to Steve and me. I hope that from wherever he is looking down at us, he is proud of our now family of four. Cheering us on with a coffee cup in hand.

I felt that Mom now had a new task to look forward to, and that was to help with the new baby. She went from grieving to a sense of purpose all within one year. But as she stayed with us, I continued to notice things that my dad had spoken about: her memory issues. Little bits and pieces that I am trying to keep track of, while at the same time taking care of my new family. I had joined the sandwich generation.

The Phone Calls, 2008

Over the next year I continue to be updated by my mom's friends on how she is doing in Starbuck. She has a wonderful core group of friends who surround her with love and assistance. They also start to notice things that I don't see because I live two hours away. I am picking up that she is starting to become repetitive. She tells me about her church meeting and then two minutes later starts to tell me the same story. I gently remind her that she has already told me the story, and she moves on to another subject.

Many of the calls I'm starting to get are about her not eating or just eating toast and cheese. Her best friend, Marilyn, called me almost monthly after my dad died and would give me an update. "She's not eating." "She could not write out her check correctly!" "Someone had to point out the way home after she went grocery shopping!" All her friends are helping me, and I'm trying to figure out a game plan for her.

One Sunday I get a call from Lois, the church secretary. She stated that she might have something of Mom's and I am confused as to what she may have.

She stated that Mom's friend Ardis had watched Mom put something into the church offering and wasn't quite sure what it was. She watched Mom dig in her favorite purse and put strange coins in the offering plate. She said she would save them for me for the next time I visited.

The very next week I was going to pick up Mom for a visit at my house, so I stopped by the church. There in an envelope were my dad's old silver-dollar Morgan coins that he had saved for a long time.

For as long as I can remember, my dad collected coins. They were kept in an old pink glass jar and we were told not to play with them. They were an instant magnet for me, just because my dad said I could not play with them. When I was little, I'd go in my room, shut the door and put them in chronological order. I loved those old coins. I had forgotten about their existence.

When Lois checked the offering, I'm sure those battered old coins stood out and she knew they were my mom's. Mom probably forgot about those coins but maybe found them again and needed some "offering" and grabbed them. My concern was that she had forgotten how important and valuable those coins were. I'm sure the church would have been thrilled to receive them.

Such is life in a small town. Old coins. Faith. Trust. And a wonderful helper named Lois. Lois would help our family out twice in a one-year span.

The Purse

If you knew my mom, you'd know it was a rare moment that she did not have a purse with her. When I would drive to Starbuck to see her and we'd run some errands, her first comment to me was "Where is my purse?" Normally it was found right by her bed or by her chair. That purse could tell some stories.

When I worked in an office building, a photographer moved downstairs. I loved his work and he used Sophia in some of his ads and marketing. One night, he brought up a purse he had made with Sophia's image on it. I thought, "Mom is going to love this!" He had me hook, line, and sinker. I didn't ask the cost. The cost will always be a secret because it didn't matter. I knew it was the best gift for Mom.

I don't remember when I gave it to her; it might have been for her birthday. But I know she had the biggest smile on her face and instantly ditched her blue fake-leather purse for her new one. Her only granddaughter at the time was now on display on her arm each time she left the house. It's funny when I think of it. I never once wanted the purse for myself, just for Mom.

The purse has been through a lot. The winter before my dad died, they vacationed in Yuma, Arizona. Dad called me to say that Mom had started to forget her purse at places they would go. He sounded frustrated with her and I could tell that this was maybe the start of her memory loss. He was not very patient with her and I was not patient with my dad. I also covered for her because I had forgotten my own purse a time or two. In full disclosure, a month after he told me about her forgetfulness, I had forgotten my own purse at home, three days in a row. THREE DAYS! My tendency to cover for her was great. My dad was starting to worry, and I was covering for her as only a daughter will do.

One morning, I called her to see how she was doing. In mid-conversation, she casually stated that she couldn't find her purse. I asked if she had looked in all her normal spots. She had. I called her friends Marilyn, Ardis, and Joyce to see if they could go to her house and look for it. They could not find it anywhere. She lives in a small town and I wasn't terribly worried, knowing that it would show up somewhere.

Day two, day three, day four . . . no purse. I started to panic since I realized she had her checkbook and all her cards (Social Security, medical numbers, license) in there. I now realized I should have taken them out and put them in a safe spot. I also realized that I had failed her a little. I wrestled with the decision to let her keep her checkbook. She would write only a few checks a month. I started to help pay for the rest of her bills when I visited her. There was part of me that did not want to take away her checkbook. I wonder if my dad had known this and took over her finances?

I think it's like taking away someone's driver's license. It simply came down to independence for her. I don't know why I kept those important cards in her purse.

I spent the whole day calling every friend and spot she had been to. I called The Water's Edge, Tom's Food Pride, Fron Church, Bremer Bank, and Samuelson's Drug Store. No purse. I even spoke to Lois at church, who had just found my mom's coins. No luck.

Day five and Lois called me from church. She gave me the good news that they had checked again in the pew and it was tucked right under it. Everything was intact, and nothing was missing. It was found at church in my beautiful small town where everyone knows whose purse it was.

The purse has been on vacations with her, witnessed a second grandchild being born, been held close to her arm when she buried her husband, been forgotten a time or two, and accompanied her on the start of her memory loss. She didn't know this yet, but it would move with her from her own home, to an assisted living home and finally to a memory care home. When I went through her purse, I could tell she was not using it the way she used to. It was dirty, and the bottom was covered with some mints, spare change, a pen, dental floss, and a few pictures of my girls. I took her checkbook and cards and hid them in my desk.

The Drive

One of the hard things that I experience as a home care nurse is family concerns about a loved one's driving abilities. "When should my parents stop driving?" or "Can you talk to them about not driving anymore?" It's a topic that can be uncomfortable for everyone involved and normally leads to hurt feelings. I think that one of the last things the elderly have regarding their independence is their ability to drive.

If I look back on the start of her memory loss, I think my greatest guilt is allowing Mom to drive when I should have stopped her sooner. When I say guilt, it really means stupidity. I hate reporting people that I feel should not drive anymore. I know that ethically and legally I must do it, but it's difficult telling them that they need to be assessed for a driving test. Normally they say, "Who are you to say that I can't drive anymore?" Even though they have no clue what they had for lunch, missed medications three days in a row, and think you are their mother.

Years ago, I took care of an attorney who was in his eighties and dying of lung cancer. For months, he would ask me if he could drive. I kept putting him off. Finally, I set up a driver's test at Courage Center. I knew he would fail and would stop asking me the same question on every nursing visit.

Fast-forward a week and I get a call from him in my office. He passed. I could tell he was over the moon. Courage Center would allow him to use his oxygen tank in the car, and his report stated that he needed a little help with his seat belt. Do you know what else? He never drove again. He just wanted to show me that he could do it. He died shortly after that. I still smile when I think of him.

I knew that Mom was still driving short distances in her small town, and she continued to make trips to see me, her girls, and her sister Gloria. She used Highway 55, a slower, more-direct route than the busy 94 freeway. My dad normally took that route, and I know they had their favorite stops along the way.

One day Mom called me from her house to let me know she was on her way for the weekend. I reminded her to call me at my office when she arrived at my house. I was at work and wasn't looking at the time. I must have gotten busy and neglected to notice that she was running really late. The office phone rang. The Crystal Police. They asked if I was Jodi. They did not sound happy.

Mom had gotten turned around and bypassed my house in Plymouth and ended up at the Target in Crystal, about five miles away. She kept telling people in Target that she was looking for her daughter, and a worried woman called the police. They arrived, and she kept showing them my work business card. Jodi Melsness, RN. I can feel the guilt and sadness, knowing that she most likely needed to stop driving. What got to me more than that, though, was the tone of contempt and anger of the male police officer on the phone.

I told work I needed to leave for a while, drove to Target and had Mom follow me to the office. Then I drove her to my house. She kept stating how sorry she was for getting turned around. She kept looking out the window with disgust with herself. I reminded her that it was all right and we would talk about it when we got home.

When we got home, we sat on the couch and I told her it might be safer for my brother to take the van, since he did not have a vehicle. She seemed accepting of this since it would be going to my brother and she felt she would be helping him.

I think she also was aware that it was time for her to stop driving. A few months after she stopped, I heard from a man who'd been helping Mom with getting gas in the van. She had no clue how to gas up her own vehicle after Dad died and he was kind enough to help her. My dad had always done this small task for her. I'm glad taking away the van went well because I know from experience that it doesn't always go this way.

Every time I drive past that Target, I think of that police officer and him staring at my name tag and looking up at my face. "She shouldn't be driving anymore." Point taken.

Years later, when she entered the memory care unit, Mom asked if she would ever be able to drive again. The loving-daughter part of me wanted to just take her in our cul-de-sac and let her drive slowly around. I did come to my senses, but the thought was there. After she stopped driving, she became the best passenger. I continued to remind her of this when we went on long trips together.

The Negotiator, June 2009

I'm sitting on the couch in our sunroom and my eyes are closed. I have just hung up the phone with Mom's best friend, Marilyn, and the news is not what I want to hear. Whenever I hear Marilyn's voice or read her emails, I get the sense that she feels I need to do more. I express that feeling to her and she responds by saying that she, and others, feels it's time that I move Mom. She knows how much I love her, but she needs to tell me these things so I can make some decisions.

Whenever I call Mom, which is mainly at night, so she can talk to her girls, she states that everything is "fine."

"Mom, how are you sleeping?" Fine.

"Mom, how did lunch with your friends go?" Fine.

"Mom, how did the walk to Dairy Queen go?" Fine.

"Mom, did you take your pills today?" Yes, I think so.

Mom neglects to tell me that her checkbook has been goofed up, so Jen from Bremer Bank called me at home and I had to intervene. I told Jen I would move some funds around and balance her checkbook when I saw her next week.

Mom neglects to tell me she forgot to pay some bills and I found the untouched mail hidden in a stack of books. I spent one whole day setting up her bills on auto-pay so she would not get overdraft fees again.

Mom neglects to tell me that after walking to Dairy Queen and back, she stopped by Tom's Food Pride to ask a stranger how to get back to her home. A neighbor of hers overheard the conversation and gave her a ride home, two whole blocks away.

Mom continues to think she is fine to stay at home and tells me that Ross, my brother, has been checking on her and not to worry. I can tell when I talk to my brother that he is just as concerned as I am. I told Ross that I was thinking of moving her to Holly Ridge, our assisted living facility in Starbuck, so I know that someone will be looking after her daily. His response to me was "You're the nurse." I would hear that phrase many times over the next eight years. You're the nurse. As if I have the magical answers to everything and I can fix all the problems with my magic nurse wand. On my day off, I call Holly Ridge. They know who I am and who my mom is. I can tell they have heard about my mom and think, "Boy, it took her a long time to call us." I now know that Marilyn had given them a heads-up and asked them to help me with the transition. There is a waiting list for Holly Ridge and my mom is twenty-two on the list.

I am now on a mission to get her placed. I email my friend Heidi, who works at the Starbuck nursing home, which is tied in with Holly Ridge, and ask for her assistance. I tell her I am grateful for whatever help she can provide and promise to stop in there when I am home next.

Meanwhile, I must be patient and wait. I have broached the subject with Mom a few times. "Mom, how would you feel if I moved you into a nice apartment at Holly Ridge? I've heard it's a nice place, and since you're no longer driving, they have a van to take you places. They even have activities like bingo, and church services. And I know you know some people who work there." Not one word from her. I can't tell if she didn't hear me or if she is ignoring what I told her. "Mom, did you hear me?" I again repeat what I just asked her, waiting for a response. She finally responds, "Why would I want to move from my house?"

I'm ready for that question. I get asked that question all the time at my job. No one feels it's a good time to move from home.

It's rare that I have a person say, "Hey, I think it's time I moved to assisted living or the nursing home!" Normally there is a fall or a broken hip that precipitates the decision.

I explain to Mom my worries about her staying in her home. "I know that Ross checks on you but not that often. You have lost some weight. Your friends are worried that you aren't eating as much as you used to, and I really want you in a more social environment. If Ruby, Joyce, Ardis, or Marilyn don't come to the house and bring you somewhere, you just sit at home alone. I want you to find something smaller and enjoy life more." I also add that Ross agrees with my idea. Remember, I am the nurse.

Mom asks, "Ross thinks it's OK?" I remind her that he does and that we can tour the apartments anytime. I tell her that we are on a wait list and she becomes suspicious. "Have you already talked to someone?" I'm now scrambling a little, but I told her that I spoke to Marilyn about the thought of moving her and that she was all for it. I can tell she's not quite sure of the idea of moving. Over the course of two months I have the same conversation with her over and over so that when we do get the call to move, she will be prepared.

On August 17, Marilyn emails me to tell me there finally is an opening. I immediately call and speak to the director at Holly Ridge. She says that Mom is still on the wait list. I'm confused, and I call Marilyn directly and she tells me that the staff is wrong, and that Mom is on the list for the next room. I'm not sure how Mom got bumped up so quickly, but sometimes it's important not to ask questions.

I call Mom the next day and tell her that she can move into her new apartment on October 1. I'm trying to be as gentle and soft as I can because I can tell this is not what she wants. "Do I have a say in moving?" I knew this question was coming. I had asked my work friends about what to do when she asks me this question. They all agree that I should tell her this move is not only for her own well-being but for mine. I remind Mom how much I worry about her being in that house alone and that I will see her just as much as before. That we will continue to travel like we have. And that she will really enjoy being around people and the number of activities. I can tell she is sad and feeling defeated all in one. I feel like a bully making her move, even though I know it's the best thing for her. I also feel guilty and overwhelmed.

Steve and I had thought about having her move in with us, possibly adding onto our house to accommodate her. I talked to her friends about it and they all agreed that Starbuck was the place to be for now and, if she gets any worse, we all could decide on where to place her next. She still knew her faithful friends. Her church was there, which she had been a part of for so many years. She loved the Dairy Queen there, which she frequented almost weekly if she could get a ride. My brother was about twenty minutes away and my dad was buried in our Lutheran cemetery plot. It was important for her to visit his grave when we were home.

We sign the papers on September 25. I briefly go through the paperwork with her because she is overwhelmed. Ross and I had become her power of attorney shortly after my dad died. I read all the necessary papers and tell her where to sign. She looks at me with anger and sadness and says more than once, "I hope you know what you are doing." That phrase would continue to roll through my brain for the next year. Do I know what I am doing? I have no idea what I am doing, even though "I am the nurse."

PART TWO

Assisted Living, 2009–2012

The Apartment

It's a beautiful fall day when we move Mom out of the home she has lived in for twenty-five years and into her new life. The week before the move, she and I discussed what would be important for her to take to her new apartment; the rest we could leave since we had no plans to sell the house yet.

Mom wants to make sure she can bring her twin bed and her dining-room set. It's an old set, but it's something she loves, so we move it, along with her couch and end tables that have seen better days. She wants to make sure I grab her bookcase along with all her books and "Don't forget the girls' pictures!"

The first time we tour her new apartment, she says she likes that she has a deck. It overlooks the school and I remind her how much time Ross and I spent playing activities there over the years. There's room for a garden, and we talk about what we could plant there.

She wanders through and inspects apartment 109. There's a cute kitchen area. She inspects the microwave, moves the chairs by the table, and opens her closet to see her coats hung up neatly and her vacuum sitting off to the side. She opens the door of her room and sees that outside is a little porch I tell her we could decorate however she wants. I say we could put a chair there if she wants to. She becomes unusually quiet.

We start to walk down the hallway to see where the washer and dryer is kept and we run into Jim Erickson, my old bus driver. He is in an apartment right by the pool table. We look at all the beautiful pictures on the wall. Mom is still quiet and I know she is adjusting to her new life. I show her how to run the washer and dryer. Residents start coming down the hallway because it's time for lunch, and she sees some people she knows. I can tell this perks her up. "Since I'm here I might as well have some lunch," she says. She gives me a tiny bit of a smile. Her placemat has her name on it already: Jeanne Lundell.

While she is eating, she watches us bring all her items in, all the ones she has requested. She is talking to her table mate but I can't tell what she is saying. I choose not to interrupt because I most likely don't want to know what she is saying. I can imagine, "My kids think this is the best place for me." "They didn't really give me a choice; just told me I'm moving here!" "Jodi is a nurse; she knows best." I can feel a headache coming on and it is only early afternoon. I wish Starbuck had an actual Starbucks coffee house. I really could use one now.

We finish getting Mom settled in. Sophia and I head to Tom's Food Pride to grocery shop for her. We see old friends, chat with the butcher, and get more for Mom than she needs. Now that her place is smaller, maybe she'll get bored and look in her fridge and see all the good things I have bought for her. Her favorite yogurts, maple pecan ice cream, easy frozen meals, fresh fruit, cheese in a variety of flavors, bananas, and her favorite snack, Snickers bars. I buy the mini Snickers in a bag and a few large ones for her purse. We spend nearly $50 and I feel she's set until the next time I see her. She casually asks me how much I spent and I'm honest with her. She gives me a shocked look and says she has never spent that much on groceries. Now if she will only start to eat the food I have purchased for her.

We are almost done with the move when Steve calls to check in on Emme and his mom, Jean. She is helping us by watching Emme. In the middle of the conversation, she casually tells Steve that Emme fell off the back of the couch and won't let Jean touch her.

When it rains, it pours. We need to leave for Minneapolis immediately and find out what is going on with Emme. Jean sounds concerned, and my fear and stress are at an all-time high.

I tell Mom that Emme has fallen but I try to make it sound like it's not a big deal. It's not the way I wanted the day to end, but I don't have a choice. I remind her that I will be back in a week and will finish setting up her pills. I also remind her that her phone is now working so she can call me later, and there is roasted chicken in the fridge. I have set up breakfast and lunch for her meal plan, and for supper she is on her own.

I feel like I'm leaving my first-born child at day care. I do not want to leave her, but I know I must. I tell myself she will be fine because my friend Carol, who is my mom's best friend's daughter, and Grace, Mom's longtime friend from church, are her aides today. They are both there to help. They work at Holly Ridge regularly and I'm so happy to see them. I repeat to myself: She will be fine. But I'm not so sure about me.

We drive the two hours home and Emme is indeed in distress. She will not let us touch her and I'm sure this will become one of my longest days ever. We take her quickly to the ER, where the staff ask me questions I cannot answer. How did it happen? Who was with her? How long has she been like this? When did she eat last? I cannot answer these questions and, as you can guess, I start to cry in front of the surprised nurse. I'm not sure if I am crying for Mom, Emme, or myself. I do not tell her I'm a nurse because I'm embarrassed we are in this situation and I was not there when it happened. I know that accidents happen and it will not be the first or last time I feel guilt for not being there, but I still feel this way.

Emme finally stops crying after the doctor examines her. She only has a bruised arm and we are relieved. We finally get home after 10 p.m. and we reassure Steve's mom that Emme will be all right. An excruciating day for our family. In hindsight, this is only preparing me for what was to come.

The Monthly Visits

Over the next three years I continue to travel four hours, round trip, to visit Mom in Starbuck. In a good month, I can see her twice. But as the months fly by, I start to see her once a month. My job as director of nursing is busy, my girls are starting school, and my life is a chaotic mess.

I try to schedule my visits with her on my days off, which are Wednesdays and Thursdays, and look at my busy calendar to try to pick the better day of the two. Because of the long drive, I arrange care for Emme with our beloved day care provider, Sue. I also get Sophia on the bus, hoping nothing goes wrong at Mom's so I can be back at 4 p.m. to get her off the bus.

I have a running list of things I need to get done. If I'm lucky, I can arrive by 11:20 a.m. and leave by 2 p.m. with all the tasks completed. Here is what I do almost every visit with Mom:

- Pick up medication at Samuelson's Drug Store.

- Check her house to make sure everything looks okay.

- Check Mom's grocery supply and make a list with her. She doesn't think she needs anything except butter pecan ice cream, Snickers, and coffee. "Oh, and white bread and any kind of cheese, please!"

- Review, organize, and pay all bills for her.

- Try to read her handwriting.

- Go to the bank and fix errors for her because I continue to let her write checks for The Water's Edge, Fron Church, and magazine orders.

- Grocery-shop. I almost always get behind because I run into people I know and they ask how Mom is doing.

- Start her laundry because she has no interest in doing it if it isn't her own machine. She is also unhappy because I'm doing her laundry, but she refuses to do it on her own. Every time I arrive, there is a big load of laundry waiting for me in her white bucket with Jeanne Lundell written on it.

- We make time for the Starbuck Dairy Queen. Snickers Blizzard or a crunch cone.

- I check in with the nursing staff to see how she is doing. I talk to Carol and Grace, her aides, and LuAnn, the director.

- Last, I set up her medications. I know them by heart and I could probably do them in my sleep. I try to set up for a month's worth of Aricept, Calcium, Celexa, Detrol, HCTZ, Lopressor, Multivitamin, Occuvite, Prilosec, Trazadone, Vitamin E, and Namenda.

To me, as a nurse in general and as her own private nurse, it is hardly anything compared to the medications I set up sometimes for my home care clients. She complains there are too many and I tell her it could be worse. We have the same conversation, every single month for three years: "Do you know that I take too many pills?!"

Every time I leave to go home, she wants me to stay longer. I feel torn between my own family of four, pressing commitments and my mother. I wonder how many people have the same feeling, this constant weight on my heart.

I feel torn telling her that I need to get back to pick up Emme and that I'm running late. I need to call my neighbor Mary and ask if she can now get Sophia off the bus. I feel torn knowing that I should have grocery-shopped myself and returned emails, and I know that the next day will be a busy workday with my own home care clients.

I am constantly torn and I will continue to feel this way every day. Every single day.

The Neurologist

Dr. Heiring,

Mom and I are coming for an appointment on Friday and I just wanted to give you a little heads-up about her. Here are a few of my concerns:

1. She is forgetting to take her pills. I know because I set them up for her every three to four weeks. I put the date on my calendar for when I need to set them up again. Last week, she still had a week left. I have noted that on two occasions. I try to call her every morning and night and she says that she has taken them.

2. She isn't reading anymore. I asked her if her eyes are bothering her, but she says no and that she just goes to bed. She has always read before bed.

3. I don't think the Namenda is helping anymore, plus it is very costly for her. She has been on Aricept for a while and I wonder if we can just keep the Aricept for her. I will bring in a copy of her medications. That is the only new medication we added. She has been having many bowel movements and I am not sure if that has something to do with it.

4. She has been in assisted living since October and has gained weight. It is hard to be two hours away from her and try to manage everything. She is not getting

any services since she has been all right on her own. She stays with me for a week once a month.

5. Can we get a weight on her when we come in to see you?

6. Please let me know what else I can do for her. We are planning our annual trip again this summer and I hope she is up to it. We did the Alzheimer's Walk last year and she was much slower in walking. Walking has always been a part of her day and now she is limited. Thank you for your time.

Jodi Melsness, RN, daughter of Jeanne Lundell

Today I am sitting with Mom on her deck and having a much-rehearsed conversation about why we have to sell her home now that she has moved to Holly Ridge. I notice that she is not listening to me, quietly watching the birds and squirrels moving from tree to tree. She leans over and whispers that our favorite old oak tree, close to her deck, survived the storm two weeks ago. I feel there is a metaphor for life somewhere in those few words.

The Fracture, 2011

On one of the coldest December days of the year, I receive a call from Carol, Mom's aide, who tells me she has fallen in her apartment. Mom did not come out for dinner and when they went to check on her, they found her on the ground with her favorite pink pajama bottoms twisted around her legs.

She was apparently tired and told the staff she was getting ready for bed, not realizing it was time for dinner. When I now think back on it, getting ready for bed was her way to escape us and herself. I felt she wanted to escape from people around her and her own confusion. In bed, she doesn't have to answer questions, make comments, or give wrong answers. She is alone with her thoughts and feelings. I know that she was starting to become aware of her confusion and memory loss and that it bothered her.

It is now about 8 p.m. and they have called 911 and are bringing her via ambulance to the hospital. I call Ross to see if he can get over there quickly. It will take me two hours to drive to Starbuck, but he is only thirty minutes away.

I receive a call from a nurse at Glacial Ridge Hospital saying Mom has fractured her left arm. I am thankful it is not her hip or even her leg, which would set her back tremendously. She is also not happy that she had to leave the assisted living facility to be evaluated. She keeps stating that she is "fine," a word that I am becoming familiar with. The nurse says she is "not fine" and that she is in visible pain and holding her left arm.

They also let me know she does not need surgery, but she will need a sling for about four weeks. I'm happy to hear this news and thankful she doesn't need to stay long in the emergency room. I can overhear her on the phone, "Call my daughter right away!" I ask them if I can talk to her and she tells me about getting on her pajama bottoms and tipping right over. At times, there is so much to be sad or angry about, but I picture her hiding in her apartment, getting ready for bed and tipping right over, and I get a nervous giggle. I am imagining my mom falling down but I am picturing much more. Hiding. Bed. Favorite pink pajamas. Bed. Fall.

"Make sure to call my daughter!"

My brother finally calls me late to tell me Mom is being kept overnight and she will be discharged in the morning. She must wear the sling every day, and physical therapy will start on Monday. I call the ER before I go to bed and talk to Mom and again she says, "I'm fine!" I remind her to be a good patient and that I will see her on the weekend. "You can't come tomorrow?" she asks. That feeling of being torn overtakes me. I remind Mom that Ross can be in charge until I get there. She seems to be all right with that.

I called Holly Ridge on Friday afternoon and was told she arrived without any problems. The nursing staff reviewed the new medication for pain and the sling protocol. We added care due to the fracture. She is not thrilled about the sling, the additional care, and the increased cost and that I'm not able to be with her. Holly Ridge will have paperwork for me to sign to increase the care and go through the cost. There is also talk of a walker for her. I can hardly wait to explain that to her.

My whole family decides to visit her Saturday and she is excited to see her girls. They wait on her hand and foot and I remind Mom that she still needs to walk but to wait for help because I see that she is a little tippy. She, of course, wants to continue to do things on her own. "How can I get coffee now?" I remind her to put on her light or keep her door open and she can yell for the staff. I'm not sure if that will work and am wondering if I should add more daily checks for her. I sign all the documents I need to sign plus I head to Tom's Food Pride to shop for her. The girls come with me and, as normal, the whole town of Starbuck has heard about her fall. We are in the store for a long time explaining what happened to her. I am fine with people snickering a little with the image of her fall.

Following the fall, I receive a call from the physical therapist saying that she wants to introduce a walker for Mom. The dreaded walker. The metal thing with four wheels and a seat with brakes. Both Mom and I aren't thrilled but for different reasons. Mom thinks she doesn't need the walker and refuses to use it. I question if she really needs it but also am sad that after all the miles and miles she has walked over the years, she must bring that ugly metal thing with her now. The beginning of her decline is what I'm really thinking.

Phone call at 8 p.m.:

Mom: "Jodi, I need some Kleenex right away. I'm out."

Me: "Mom, did you check the closet? I thought I left you some extras."

Puts the phone down loudly. Takes forever to return.

Mom: "I couldn't find any. Can you bring me some today?"

Me: "Mom, remember I am in Plymouth and its 8 o'clock at night. Why don't I call one of your friends to get a few boxes?"

Mom: "You could stop by the store today and pick some up."

Me: Deep breathing. "I'll call Carol or Marilyn tomorrow to get you some, Mom. Don't worry, I'll take care of it."

Mom: "No, I only want you to do it."

Me: Sigh.

The Subtle Changes

As the months go by, the staff update me on how she is doing, sometimes daily. They go through their concerns and I list my own. I worry if I am making the best decisions for her. Mom and I argue about a few things.

She is not keeping her apartment clean and I am surprised at this. "Mom, there is dust all over the place! I bought you cleaning supplies and rags, plus this would be good exercise for you! You didn't even make your bed today." My mother is the cleanest, hardest-working person you could ever know. She kept our house neat, clean, and in working order. She ironed every piece of clothing in our house and washed windows almost weekly. She has always been a cleaning force. Not anymore. I feel like I am shaming her to clean and she couldn't care less. This memory loss does not mess around. It is now affecting her ability to clean and I think she would be mortified to know this. So I add to her assisted living package a cleaning fee of $64 per month. I know this disease is bad when she is okay paying that much for cleaning. Clearly, things have changed.

I receive calls from Fron Church and Holly Ridge telling me they do not want Mom walking the four blocks to church anymore. I'm on the phone with the nursing director, LuAnn, and I feel myself almost start to cry. "Do you feel she can't do it anymore?" LuAnn agrees. I find out later that she could not find her way back from church one Sunday. One of the things I told Mom when I moved her to Holly Ridge was that she could still walk to church. I wasn't worried because she had made that quick trip so many times, she knew Starbuck so well, and she walked the whole town for miles and miles. The miles stopped after that phone call. I now needed to find people to take her to church and drop her back off at Holly Ridge. I called Ruby, Ardis, Marilyn, and Joyce, and they worked out a system for picking up my mom every Sunday. My small village continues to take care of my mother and I am thankful.

The very next week, after taking care of the walking issue, my brother's friend Jerry calls to say that my mom's mail has been backing up in her mailbox. Jerry works at our small post office and felt I needed to know. My mom loved getting her mail every single day. It was now the most she was walking every day. Fifty feet to her small box to get mail. I had a bright red string attached to her mailbox key so that it would be easy for her to find.

I called Mom right away to ask if she had gotten her mail lately. She was not sure and I told her to look in her basket by the couch. "What key am I looking for?" I reminded her about the mail key with the red string on it. "It's not in the basket." I find myself deep breathing. Where is her key now? I called Holly Ridge and asked if an aide would go in Mom's room and look for her key. No key.

I send Jerry a message and ask him what I can do about the lost key. He will make another key for her mailbox and bring it up to Holly Ridge. I wasn't sure what to put on the key so she wouldn't lose it. There are so many people that have begun to help Mom and me. It's hard not to feel overwhelmed. Jerry would help us again a few months later by making us another key, but by then I have an aide start to get her mail every day. I feel I am problem-solving almost every day, from two hours away.

Over the next few weeks I'm having trouble getting up to see Mom. My nursing job has been busy, Sophia is starting to have more hockey practices, and I feel that I have been neglectful in everything. I ask my friend Carol, who works at Holly Ridge, if she will help with laundry and cleaning when I can't be there. I run it by Mom and she doesn't understand what I am trying to tell her.

I decide to hire Carol to help our family. By this time I have put almost everything on auto-pay for Mom and I can pay her bills from my computer. I still allow her to write some checks, and Jen at Bremer Bank has been wonderful at helping me figure out issues if Mom has made an error.

Mom's friends continue to take her places, look after her and let me know what is happening on a weekly basis. Marilyn emails me monthly to check in. Holly Ridge is letting me know that we need to add services. They are refusing to let me set up her medications anymore and I will now need to pay for the med service at $165 a month. I can hardly stand to pay for this since it's something I can do for her free of charge. I feel her rate going up and her expenses rising. I sign more papers and even more papers and I continue to worry about her from afar. The nurses are letting me know that she is starting to have more incontinence issues and needs more reminders with everything. Mom's phone conversations are becoming more repetitive and we talk about selling her house to help pay for care. My brother has been reluctant to sell her home and I have called my friend Lara to ask some questions about selling it. There is so much to think about and organize. I have forgotten appointments at home. I am becoming anxious and unhinged. I talk to friends, I cry with my sister-in-law, Wendy, and I start to see a wonderful counselor. She is the first person to ask me, "Why don't you bring her closer to you?" I pause for a moment and think about that. Why don't I move her closer? How come I haven't thought of that before?

The Nursing Home

I have rehearsed the conversation in my head repeatedly. I have talked to my girlfriends, spoken to my nursing co-workers and received a long email from Mom's friend Marilyn. They all say the same thing. Move her closer to her family, mainly me.

I weigh the options of keeping her in the hometown she loves or moving her, which ultimately would be easier for me. I call for prices for the Minnewaska Home and tour a total of fifteen places near my home in Plymouth. Many of the memory care units I have been in over the years of nursing. I feel like I have made a hundred calls and I keep rehearsing my talk with Mom.

I schedule a time to tour the Minnewaska nursing home in Starbuck, the one I have visited my whole life, where my childhood friend Heidi works. We talk about what it would be like to have Mom live there.

I slowly walk the halls of the nursing home I picture my Mom living in. My mind drifts to the hours I have spent there as a child, mainly singing in groups for the residents and visiting the many people that my mom continued to visit and take care of. She regularly visited people in this beautiful home, my old neighbor Muriel Aslagson, my adopted grandma, Julia Danielson, and my mom's cousin, Curt Anderson, along with countless other people. She was so devoted to this place that I am now wondering if it should be her last home.

I look in residents' rooms, taking in the smell a nursing home emits, listening to the chatter of the staff and reading a name on a door, my former school superintendent. I am surprised to see his name, wondering what had become of him. I always enjoyed and respected him and he was always very kind to me. I suddenly feel so old, seeing his name so bold on the door. I want to go in and talk to him, but I'm not sure it's appropriate; plus he's asleep in his chair. I want to tell him that I love my hometown and that I became a nurse and what I am doing here, finding a placement for Mom. I miss this slower life. I then walk onto the memory care unit.

The doors open and I can feel the change. I immediately note the noise level. Someone is banging on a table. I am home in a way, having spent four years in a memory care unit when I was a nursing assistant in the early nineties. I walk around noting the interaction and see an older woman sitting in a chair. I see the name above her door and realize she is my mom's old boss. She has aged so much and I realize she is the one doing the rhythmic banging on the table. I kneel to get on her level, give her a big smile and tell her, "Hello!" She has drool coming from her mouth and her hair is a mess. When my mom used to work at her store, she was one of the best-dressed people I knew. I always admired her style and her hair, which was always perfectly in place. She was incredibly kind when I stopped in to see Mom. Her husband was just as kind.

Now when I look at her, I am saddened. This disease has taken her too and I wonder if she is one of the people my mom would come to see on a regular basis. She is trying to tell me something and her words are coming out in a jumbled mess. The banging. The yelling. The noise overall. I can't have Mom live in this place, knowing that she still knows me, my girls, and her family. She will hate me. She has always been sensitive to noise and still has the hearing of a hawk. Her brain may be slowly deteriorating but the noise level will drive her insane. I know I can't continue to make the four-hour round-trip drive and I know that she will end up in this unit. I can feel tears building. I must move her near me or have her live with us. I know this building was so important to her life, but I am choosing to move her to Minneapolis. And I continue to make choices for my mother and I wonder if I'm doing the right thing.

I receive an email from my childhood friend Sarah after a very long week:

Jodi,

I'm so sorry. It is so, so hard to make sense of it all. Cry if you need to, and remember that each day is a new day. You can only do so much, and it's okay. Your burden is big right now and it's okay that you can't do it all. No one can. Sometimes, wearing matching socks makes the day a success. You are doing amazing things by having your mom around your girls—they will have memories, and your mom, on some level, knows how hard you're working to do it all. I know she does. It is heartbreaking to watch, and it's important to remember that each day is a new day. Tomorrow you'll get a different glimpse into what is going on with her mind, and you might get a nugget that you'll carry with you forever.

The last time I saw my dad before he died, he rambled on and on, and then he said, "Gee, you're pretty!" And then he rambled on and on some more. He then said, "You should take a trip!" Which just makes me cry, because he knows how much I love to travel. It felt like he was talking to me, even though he wasn't "all there." Your mom will have moments like that too. You just have to hold out hope that they'll happen.

Hang in there. I'm thinking about you and hoping that tomorrow is easier. Remember that crying is okay! It's hard and sometimes you just have to let it out.

Take care,
Sarah

Sarah's father, Chuck, was our attorney in Starbuck. He retired from his law practice and was showing signs of dementia. Sarah's mom took care of him at home and they eventually moved him to a nursing home.

I keep this note on my special board near my desk. I read it often for encouragement. This is an example of the village of people starting to help me.

The Love Story

I was going through Mom's stuff and trying to decide what to keep and what to toss. It was a difficult task for me.

While looking through her journals and boxes, I found this picture in a very old book, along with some other special pictures. It's my first picture and on the back, in my mom's handwriting, it states, "Taken January 14th, 1970, the day we adopted Jodi." If you look closely, you will find there is a smirk on my face and you will note that I was well fed at Lutheran Social Services. It is a picture that has long been forgotten but was very important to Mom. It marks the day that both Mom and Dad welcomed me into their family. My brother, Ross, is almost three in this picture. He, of course, came first.

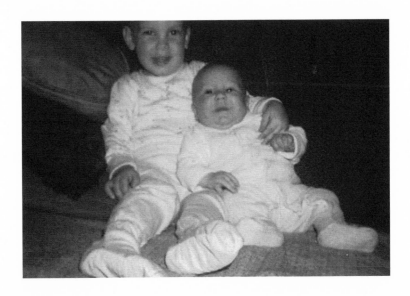

Both my parents were young (twenty) when they got married just after World War II. Life was good for them and they enjoyed traveling and had many adventures together. For over twenty years, they tried to have children. When Mom was young, she had minor surgery and they think that's the reason she couldn't conceive. It is such a different world now and I imagine if she were young today she would be able to conceive. It's difficult for me to imagine their sadness of not being able to get pregnant. They chose Plan B.

Ross and I were both adopted through Lutheran Social Services (LSS). In the process, they had highs and lows. Back then, you could not have any drug/alcohol problems and you really needed to be perfect. My dad struggled with alcohol and with staying sober. LSS denied them at first. My dad had also set up a savings account for the future Baby Lundell, and a social worker at LSS felt my dad was "materialistic" and denied them once again. It was difficult for them, but in 1967 they got a baby boy. As the story goes, Ross picked out a brown-eyed girl, two and a half years later, to be his sister. It is a fact that he has wanted to give me back ever since.

After I was adopted, we moved from Plymouth to a wonderful small town, surrounded by farmland and a beautiful lake. It was a perfect place to raise children and we grew up knowing we were loved. As in any family, there were ups and downs. But as communities go, Starbuck was ideal.

I look at this picture now and I am so thankful for the person who made the difficult choice of giving up a baby and letting someone else give her a better life. How unselfish of her to decide that she or her family was unable to raise me and love me enough and give me away to parents that really wanted children. That is the ultimate love story.

As Mom starts to walk in this fog of Alzheimer's disease, I know how much we were wanted and loved, the same feeling I'm sure she felt that day in January. When we were driving to Starbuck a few years ago, I asked if she was sad that she never got to experience birth. Her response was that she never had to go through any labor pain and that LSS just handed her a clean, happy baby. She reminded me that I caused her other pain, which made me laugh.

Life is all about choices. I am thankful for the woman in Minneapolis who gave my parents much happiness.

The House Sale, 2011

My parents' home has been sold to someone my family knows. I'm thrilled it has sold, but I confess it has been the most stressful time since my dad passed away.

The house, which used to be Starbuck's old mortuary, has been a home to our family since I was sixteen. It's centrally located to everything, two blocks from the hardware store and the grocery store with the church right across the street. In our small town there is really everything you could need within a one-mile radius. The bank, clinic, school, Dairy Queen, gas station, church, and restaurant, all on the edge of a beautiful lake called Minnewaska, which is Minnesota's thirteenth-largest lake. This small town and home have been important to our family and there is a lot of grief in selling it.

As I look around the two-story home, the one my dad added onto and restored, I have such happy memories. All the celebrations, the holidays, the activities, and friends that have passed through the old brown door. All the hours spent mowing the never-quite-green lawn with the steep bank and sitting on the large rock in our front yard.

I spent time picking strawberries in our garden and harvesting rhubarb from the plants that they had moved from the farm. I look at the rhubarb plants and see the plant that was stolen. Years ago, when I was in college, my dad called me one morning to let me know that someone had dug up one of his plants in the middle of the night and left a huge, gaping hole where their beloved rhubarb should have been. He was angry and appalled that someone would have the nerve to dig up a plant right underneath his nose. My parents were very generous, as I think all people in small towns are, and I know that if someone had asked for some rhubarb, my parents would have happily shared their supply with them. Instead, The Rhubarb Thief, as my dad liked to call him, took something from them and ruined their line of rhubarb. The thief took the second one in, not even the end rhubarb plant, which I think enraged my engineer dad even more. To this day, we never found out who took their rhubarb.

My friend Lara has been helping me with the sale of the house. When the house was appraised, we found some surprising things. First was that our upstairs bathroom had been completely shut off. There was no water, and my dad had done something to the pipes that left us needing to make repairs. My brother was not very happy with this since he felt the sale needed to be as is. We had many conversations with Lara about this problem. The second thing is that the appraiser had found evidence of bats in our attic. Yes, bats.

When I would come home from Minneapolis, my mom would tell me she killed another bat with a tennis racket. She took great pride in letting us know that SHE had killed the bat, not my dad. Occasionally, I would find a dead one on the stairs going up to my bedroom.

Before the sale could be complete, I had to spend hours tracking down an exterminator. I called places to get quotes and the prices were high, plus they charged for mileage. I also had to talk with Ross and try to explain why we must spend this amount of money on the house. Costs were starting to add up, but we didn't really have a choice if we were to sell the house. We needed to fix the bathroom and get rid of the bats.

While the exterminators were in the attic, they found my dad's green typewriter. They pulled it out and it was full of bat feces and dust. I put gloves on, cleaned it up, put in some paper, and it worked! The typewriter was a symbol of my dad and all his typewritten letters to me. When he would write me after I left high school, he would either type me a letter or handwrite one in neat, blocked handwriting. If I received a handwritten letter, I knew I was in trouble. When I had done something that did not meet his approval, he would get out his pencil or pen and draft me a letter that would tell me he knew better and so should I. If I received a letter typewritten on his heavy old Royal, it would be of fatherly advice. Maybe I didn't do something correctly but if I did it this way, the results would be better. Messages of wisdom lovingly typed one finger at a time, on paper for me to see.

Steve and I start to clean out my parents' home. We find remarkable things.

- Hundreds of vases stacked away in cupboards; short, tall, skinny, large. My mom was a vase hoarder. From all the flowers I have bought her for twenty-plus years, she kept the vase.

- Sewing needles, hundreds of different kinds of thread, hundreds of quilting blocks, and McCall's patterns that date back to the sixties. She took great pride in sewing matching outfits for Ross and me. I have the pictures for proof.

- She saved every program from every school event I ever attended and some that I did not attend. Boxes of choir concert pictures and programs, all my sporting event clippings from the *Starbuck Times*, medals, perfect-attendance awards, church programs of plays. She saved it all, including my wedding items and all the pictures I have sent her of my girls.

- Five sets of dishes, all in a different pattern. Many of them I had never seen her use before, still in their boxes.

- Hundreds of Tupperware items with *Lundell* written on the bottom in black marker so that it would be returned to her after she provided a meal or dessert for a funeral or wedding at church.

- Books. I can hardly stand to pack up her books that she is not reading anymore.

- She even kept church bulletins, saved with a binder wrapped around them.

I don't know what to keep and what to throw. I am so glad my husband is here to help me. I hold up something and he says, "Toss!" Of course, he is not nostalgic for any of it; it doesn't have a history to him and I should be glad. As I watch the giant dumpster start to fill with all their items, I have to take a moment to be sad. I wonder what they would think of me tossing all their items. I have kept the important things that I want my kids to have, but I decide to donate a lot of it and I find places for the vases, her sewing items, her sewing machine, and the dish sets that must have been important to her to keep this long.

When we finally have the house clear, I realize I can't find my dad's typewriter. The house is empty so I should I be able to find it easily. I look the whole house over and I can't find it. I have come to realize that someone has thrown it in the dumpster. I again take a moment to mourn for the typewriter but, as a good husband does, Steve brings me back by saying, "Where the hell are you going to put it?" He's correct, as he normally is. Maybe it could have sat by my dad's old bowling trophy.

When the house is clear, I go back to my mom's to let her know that we finished. She thinks we are talking about the old red house in Crystal. She doesn't remember the twenty-plus years she spent in her Starbuck home with Dad.

For some reason, I am glad for that. It makes it easier that she has forgotten, though I will remember the home for the both of us. Bats and all.

I've just arrived at Mom's apartment and I see her answering machine blinking with twenty-six unheard messages. I push the button and listen to the twenty-six messages, all from MCI, her long-distance phone service. They state that she forgot to pay her last bill. The "she" part in the message would pertain to me. Mom is listening to the messages and quietly says, "I think they are mad at me."

Way to wake the sleeping bear inside of me. My first project today is calling MCI. They are going to love our conversation.

The Talk, September 2012

It's a beautiful fall day and Mom and I are sitting on the porch outside her Holly Ridge apartment. The birds are singing us a song and I am noting the dry, dead plants that I bought her this summer. On the phone I would remind her about the plants on the deck to give her a small project she could attend to. Flowers and plants were almost as much a part of her as cooking and baking.

When we lived on the farm, my mom had two big gardens for vegetables and her flowers. They were her pride and joy. For many summers, she sold raspberries from the side of the road: $1 a pint and we split the cost if I helped her on those long, warm farm days. Now as I pick off the dead leaves, I think how she would be mortified to know that she has let the plants die. She doesn't notice them and I realize I have spent a fortune on them, just to have them fade away.

Both Mom and I are sitting in her old yellow and green lawn chairs, with some of the plastic starting to crack. I give her one of the better chairs, and I bring out a pot of coffee. I want to make sure she is comfortable as I deliver my long-rehearsed speech. I've practiced with my friends, my colleagues, my counselor, and my husband. I'm about to move her again and I'm prepared for her pushback.

In the mail arrived a four-page note from the Starbuck Clinic. I reviewed all the information. What struck me was the very last part of the letter, something that made me sad. Dr. Bosl had made a clinical note at the end of his visit, a note that I am so familiar with. A summary or recap of how the visit went in which I read my own clients' notes, since I am not normally there at their appointment. It reads:

"Remembers husband died, no idea as to when or how long they were married, etc. Clearly has marked worsening of Alzheimer's over time, unlikely related to UTI alone (unable to provide specimen this a.m.). Probably needs to consider nursing home placement as is too confused to continue to function in Holly Ridge setting, has no idea where she lives, etc. Discussed with Holly Ridge staff recommendation for NH. They will contact the patient's daughter. Medical Decision Making: More than half of this 50 minutes was spent in counseling. Robert H. Bosl, MD."

I have read those words repeatedly. No one called me about this letter. The staff have been telling me she needs to move because she is becoming more incontinent and they try to explain to me that Holly Ridge is an assisted living facility.

I realize it is assisted living and I realize they have been assisting her like we have contracted, but no one tells me about this note and I am saddened that my mom's hometown doctor didn't take the time to call and let me know. I feel like I'm now really under the gun to move her, but no one wants to be honest with me. I am sure the reason is that no one wants to tell me. They just keep using the word incontinence. "We can't have her stay here."

So here we sit in the old, decaying lawn chairs and I'm ready, but she is not. She is sitting with her coffee cup in her hand and looking out over the football field and school. The old, worn football field is nostalgic for me because it's where I spent all my school years. All the nine-man football games our family attended, the dodgeball games where the girls tried to not get hit by the boys, running the mile on the black, cracked, bumpy track, and my many years of softball. I cannot begin to count how many times our family has attended sporting events, choir concerts, meetings, games, and conferences at the school. I wonder if she remembers all those happy times when she looks out her window.

"Mom, I've been thinking about a lot of things lately. I have been touring some places near my home for you and I have narrowed it down to a great place only two miles from my work and just a little farther from our house. That way I could come and see you every day and not have to drive so far. The girls are excited about having you closer, and Steve and Ross will help with everything. I think this would be the best for all of us. I've talked to Ross about it and he is all right with it."

I look at her for a reaction. She is watching the birds soaring in the sky and the fat squirrels running across the brown field.

"I have toured a place called Clare Bridge and they have some nice large apartments. They even have their own coffee room and make their own meals right on site. There is a big glass birdcage and they have activities every day, plus an exercise class. I spoke to the director and they even have a church group every Wednesday that you can attend. When I looked at rooms last week, I could smell chocolate chip cookies baking. And I forgot to tell you they have cooking classes. Doesn't that sound fun?"

I turn to look at her from my chair and she is drinking her coffee and I can tell she is ignoring me. "Mom, did you hear what I said? I'd like to move you closer to me so I can see you weekly instead of traveling so much."

She slowly asks me if I see the squirrel running across the field. "Do you see how green the tree is? It's such a pretty green." She has been obsessed with green lately. On my trips to bring her down to Minneapolis, she will talk about the tree colors for two hours and ask if I have ever seen such a pretty green tree. Over and over again.

I can feel sadness and a little bit of anger take over. "Mom, I want to move you near me. Are you all right with that?" I put her coffee cup down and turn her toward me. I can tell she wants to keep looking at the animals. I can't tell if she's purposely ignoring me or if it's just a new part of the disease. I can feel my eyes get misty and I wait quietly. The birds are singing and I'm waiting for my mother to say yes, though I'm not sure if she knows what I'm talking about.

She finally looks at me and tells me, "Whatever you feel is best, Jodi." I'm waiting for her to tell me that I'm the nurse and that I should know everything, since that's what my brother normally says. She has given me permission to move her, though I know she will most likely forget this conversation tomorrow. I hug her and tell her not to worry. I wish I could say that to myself.

The Second Move, November 2012

I've requested a few days off from work to move Mom. My husband, my brother, and I pack her up for another disruption in her life. She has long forgotten my conversation with her about moving, and she seems surprised to see Steve with me. I go with the flow. I hope the move goes much smoother than her first move. I know there aren't any bats.

I can tell she is worried and nervous, and she keeps asking us what we are doing. I remind her that we are moving her closer to me and that we agreed that it would be better so I can come and see her every day.

"Every day?"

"Every day, if I don't have something going on, Mom."

There is not as much to pack as a few years ago. Plus in her new apartment she really only needs her clothes, toiletries, some books, and the girls' pictures and albums. They are supplying her with a twin bed and a dresser. I bought some new sheets for her at Target and have washed her blue comforter. I will plan on buying a TV as soon as I get her settled, a large one so she can watch *Wheel of Fortune* and *The Price Is Right*.

It doesn't take us long to get her packed up in my SUV, her life now settled into my car. I can tell she doesn't know what is happening and why everyone is telling her goodbye. Carol, Grace, Marilyn, Ruby, Joyce, and all the residents wishing her good luck. She gives me a look like she is not interested in any of this. She holds onto a card they have signed for her.

"Goodbye, Jeanne! Keep in touch!" People are hugging her and I really want to get on the road because I need to get her settled into her new place.

I make sure she has gone to the bathroom and I grab some coffee near the nursing station for both of us. I wish the cups were bigger because I know we are both going to need it.

As we pull out of the driveway, I begin to realize that she will most likely never see her hometown again. There is a rare chance that I may come back, but I know it is unlikely. It would mean taking her out of Clare Bridge and driving a round trip of four hours. I will, if it comes to that. I decide to drive her around her cherished town. We pass by Holly Skogen, our small Scandinavian park that the girls have been to, looking for the little gnomes and trolls. We drive two blocks up to Fron Church, where she has spent years of her life singing in the choir, making meals for funerals and weddings, quilting, planning the Easter Garden, teaching Sunday school, and praying for everyone. This is the church that I was confirmed and married in. My dad even helped with the design of the new addition. We are slowly driving by for one last look.

We head up one block to the house that we just sold. We drive by her garden, the rock in the yard and her seven rhubarb plants. We pull in the driveway and the Lundell sign is gone, as is her memory of this happy home.

We drive past the Minnewaska Home where she visited so many people and where I almost placed her. We drive by all of her favorite stores. Tom's Food Pride, Isdahl's Hardware Store, The Bakery, Touch of Class, and Bremer Bank. Special places where we spent so much time. We continue to Hobo Park and past her most favorite place, Dairy Queen. We drive slowly by Starbuck Park, where we spent so much time during church in the park, Fourth of July parties, and family reunions playing horseshoes. We continue past the beach of our beautiful lake, where we spent countless hours swimming and boating, lake itch and all.

We drive through the Water's Edge parking lot. I remind her it's a restaurant that she and Dad went to many times and where she would meet her friends for lunch. She just listens to me talk and point and I know she is overwhelmed. We drive for a bit on the south shore and look at all the nice cabins and I point out the Lommens' home, which she used to clean weekly. I'm not sure if she knows what we are doing but we are saying goodbye. Or rather I'm saying goodbye for her.

We turn around and head back to town, and I point out the airport and Feigum's Nursery, where she ordered so many flowers and plants over the years. We end up at Dairy Queen and she orders her normal treat, a small Snickers Blizzard. How many times has she frequented this place and how many times has she been turned around walking but found this marker and knew where she was? It's the final stop in her goodbye and an important one. I tell her we have a Dairy Queen by our house and my work so that she won't miss her Snickers Blizzard. She gives me a quick, small smile. We are on the road now and I can feel tears while we pass the bend on our way to Glenwood. How good this town was to my mom when she needed help and how much my mom loved Starbuck.

We travel through all the same towns she has traveled through for hundreds of trips: Sauk Centre, Saint Cloud, Avon, Monticello, Elk River, Maple Grove, and Plymouth. All familiar towns but not to her anymore. She talks about the green trees (again), says I am a good driver and I need a haircut. I'm trying to prep her for her new home so that it might stay in her brain for the next half hour before we arrive. But she remains quiet.

We pull up to Clare Bridge and I'm feeling anxious. I was telling a friend that it felt like dropping my child off at a new daycare, not knowing how she will get along. Will she make new friends? Will she like the food and nap well? I sit for a second in the car and breathe deeply. I need to be strong and confident for her. And for me too. We will both be all right, I keep thinking. I can do this.

I leave all her things in the car and get her ugly metal walker out of the car. "Where are we?" she asks. "We are at Clare Bridge, your new home that I found. Remember it is right by my work and our home?"

Of course she doesn't remember. She's arriving at her new home in memory care and she doesn't remember I have told her this twenty-plus times. I'm breathing deeply. We push the button to be buzzed in and we wait for the door to open. It is a fifty-five-bed home that is locked so the residents can't wander out or "escape." You need to buzz to get in and out.

I hear the buzz that I will become used to on every visit and I tell Mom that we can go in. I hold the door. She gives me a worried look and we head in the direction of our new life.

PART THREE

Memory Care

The Adjustment

Memory care. My mom is now living in memory care. I repeat the words to my friends, my family, and myself over and over again. My mom, who has raised me for forty years, is in memory care. She is now with other people who need memory care.

The first day we arrive, I want Mom to embrace and love her new "home." She is quiet while I chat away about the amenities. "Your new place has its own beauty shop, there is a coffee nook where we can have coffee together, and they have a lovely dining room where they have really great food!" We continue to walk the halls and I point out the fish tank, the brightly colored birds in the bird aviary, the nursery, the workshop, and the dress-up room.

She is still quiet but I can tell she is intrigued by the smell of coffee and the birds. We grab a cup of coffee and I head down to her room to see if everything is ready. Her favorite bedding is in place. The pictures of all of us, especially her girls, are on the wall. I went to Best Buy last week and spent way too much on a flat-screen television for her to watch her favorites programs. It sits on her dresser. I remember the salesperson telling me that his own grandmother had memory loss and how hard it was for their family. He gave me a discount when he rang it up. I am grateful for any break I can get. I look out the window and see the new birdhouse I purchased for her, swinging on a metal stand. Birds are flocking to it and I'm happy that she'll be able to watch them. Lately, birds have brought her comfort.

I walk back to the aviary to find her watching the birds and pointing at them. Someone has given her a snack from the nook area and I can tell she is more engaged. People are so kind and welcoming. I can feel my anxiety starting to lessen. I get her up gently and put her walker in place and we head down to her room. We walk past the beauty shop and the dining hall and we look out at the patio. "Mom, we can sit out here and have dinner if you want. Look at all the plants!" She seems interested in the plants.

We arrive at her room and there is a big sign on her door in big, bold letters: "Welcome, Jeanne Lundell!!"

"Is this my new room?" She slowly walks into her new home, glancing at the chair I have moved twice now and I hope is a comfort to her. I see her look around and spot her favorite pictures and a desk that I have put her items on. She picks up the picture of my dad from her bedside table. "This is Russell?" I nod my head and show her their wedding picture on the wall, right next to the picture of Jesus in an old, worn frame, which used to be in their bedroom on the farm. I am aware that Jesus has followed her to her new home also. I hope he continues to watch over her.

Mom walks to the bed and pats her blue comforter. She reminds me that she loves the color blue. In the past few months it has been the color green. But I am all right with the switch of colors.

She walks around the large space and I show her the bathroom, her items on the left, her roommate's on the right. I have everything set up for her: nice soaps, a new toothbrush, almond shower gel, her hairbrush, and her mother's antique hand mirror. I open up the closet to show her all the things I have organized for her. I am proud of how I have helped her, but she doesn't say a word and shuts the door and walks out. She spies her chair and sits down on it. I put the foot stool up and cover her up with a blanket. I love her new room and I patiently wait for her to say something. But as I come out of the bathroom, she is sound asleep.

I see that her roommate is also sleeping, and I head out the door to bring some coffee for us. The unit is shaped like a square and I walk past the nursing station. I poke my head in to introduce myself and I meet a wonderful nurse named Amanda. I want to make sure I connect with them, like I try to do with my own clients' families. I always feel that if you are genuine and sincere and try not to drive them crazy, it will be beneficial to you both. I can tell they are busy and I walk along the hallway. I say hi to people and watch the activities that are going on. I see a group sitting in the dining room and the activity aide is reading the news to them. I'm not sure Mom will like this, but I'll ask her about it. I peek my head into the beauty shop and introduce myself to the stylist. I want to schedule a wash and cut for Mom this week if I can; she is long overdue. I like her immediately and think there is a special place in heaven for a woman who styles hair in a memory care unit. I am sure each day is new for her but I can imagine it's rewarding. I let her know that Mom has beautiful hair but it is stick straight and she likes a perm every so often. I can tell she has been doing this for a while. She thanks me for the update.

I walk back to the room and turn the TV on to wake her because it will be suppertime soon and I have scheduled to eat with her tonight. She wakes up slowly and notices I am sitting on her bed. "Where am I?" I remind her that she took a short nap and this is her new home. I remind her it is close to my house now. I can come and see her every day for the new few weeks. "Do I live here?" I point at all the pictures on the walls, her chair, and the ceramic church in the corner. I pat her bedspread and show her the bird stand outside.

"I know it will take some time to adjust, Mom, but you are so close to me now and we can come see you all the time. I made an appointment for you to get your hair done this week and the stylist is very nice." She pats her short white hair and asks if she looks bad. I let her know that she has always had it done once a week and I wanted her to still do that, so that she looks nice. She continues to stare at me and I laugh. "I want you to look nice, all right?"

We pass a nursery where there are plastic babies and puzzles. There is a baby crib and blankets and it is dimly lit. I let her know that the girls can play in there when they come and visit. She asks where they are and I remind her that they're at home with Steve and will visit her in the next few days. I say their names so that she continues to remember them. She nods as if she knows.

We sit down at a table for four, though they have moved one person so that I can sit with Mom. I have asked for her to sit with people she can converse with. One woman sitting to Mom's left is young, younger than I expect, but I know that especially in my profession, we see memory loss at all ages. She is kind and sweet and I hope Mom bonds with her.

The other woman who sits with her is quiet and eating the food in front of her. The younger woman and I chat. She likes my checkered shirt and I tell her a little about Mom. I pick up on the younger woman's loss quickly and I can tell she is gentle, a good fit for Mom.

We get done with supper and the staff hands her a warm cloth to wash her hands. She is unsure of what to do and I show her. She asks me for more coffee and I get her some. I introduce the dining room aides to Mom and hope that Mom is kind to them. I begin to feel overwhelmed because I must go soon, but I want to stay and help get Mom ready for bed.

We walk slowly back to her room and I catch her peeking into the nursery. We walk by the younger woman's room and she has already taken off her shoes and is barefoot. She wants me to see her room and I promise to come back after I get Mom ready for bed. I wonder how young her family is and how hard it must have been to make the decision to place her here. Do they feel the same worry as I? Do they worry about money, paperwork, bills, and the overall unknown with this disease? Did they worry they were making the right decisions?

I finally meet my mom's roommate when we arrive. I have heard about her and I was warned a little about her daughter, who can be overwhelming at times. Mom's roommate is nonverbal and needs help getting into bed. I tell her my name and introduce Mom but she only makes nonsensical noises. I hope it doesn't go on all night so she can't sleep. I know Mom's favorite place is bed and I would hate if that disturbed her.

I wait for the staff to get the roommate ready for bed and try to stay out of the way. The room they share is fairly large and there is no curtain to separate them. Mom and I watch *Wheel of Fortune* and I feel I need to check on my own family. The staff is sweet to Mom and I let them know that I can get her ready for bed. They seem surprised and explain that it's their job, but I let them know that I used to be an aide, not sharing yet that I'm a nurse. I told them I get Mom ready for bed all the time, and one of them seems relieved. I know how hard many of them work and to have one less resident is helpful.

I bring Mom to the bathroom and run warm water in the sink. She does her business and gets her warm, fluffy pink pajamas out. Her eyes light up and I know she likes them. I get her washed up, help her put them on, and then get her toothbrush ready. She gives me a look and I know she feels bad that she has forgotten this simple step. I hope the staff help her. I worry.

I put nice-smelling lotion on her and we shuffle off to bed. She notices the blue comforter and lets me know that she has one like that at home. I tell her that it is hers from home and she appears confused. I try to keep things simple for her. Simple statements. Simple conversations. Nothing too detailed.

I shut her new TV off and help her into her twin bed with her blue comforter. I know she is tired. We have had a long day driving, moving, adjusting, and hoping. Well, that would be me: hoping that she will adjust to her new home and roommate, adjust to the staff, the food, and a new change in her life. Maybe she won't remember all of these changes? I wonder what she is really thinking and if it is just a jumbled mess of nerves, matter, neurons, and cells misfiring in her brain?

I lean over to kiss her and her eyes are already closing. I can hear her roommate mumble and I hope it doesn't bother Mom's sleep. "I love you, Mom. Sleep well!" I move my dad's picture close to her so if she wakes up, it will be right beside her. I also move my picture closer, hoping that she will never forget my face.

I turn the lights off and leave the door open a crack. I have left the bathroom light on in case she gets up and wonders where the bathroom is. I hope they check on her at night. I hope they take good care of her. I hope she sleeps well. I continue to feel like this is my child instead of my mother.

I walk out and gently knock on the nurses' station door and I thank the staff. I ask if they will check on her more often tonight since she is new, and they assure me they will.

I walk to the entrance. I will walk through these doors hundreds of times, with the same buzzing sound. Letting me out into the world that doesn't include my mother. She is in a memory care unit.

I get in my car and I can feel how exhausted I am. I feel tense and anxious with such sadness. I look up and watch a couple walking on the sidewalk. Not a care in the world. They have no idea that Mom was a walker too and that if she didn't have this disease, she and I would be walking and we would not be here. I can feel tears start to fall. I feel so unsure. Is this the best place for her? What happens if she hates it here? I feel like I am abandoning her with strangers. She doesn't know a soul. What would my dad think, staring back at me from Mom's bedside table? My dad would say to do what is best for her. I'm trying, Dad. I'm trying.

I start the car and head home to my family.

The Winter, January 2013

My mom has been in Clare Bridge for two months and she has adjusted well. For two weeks straight I see her every day. In my own work, I know how hard it is to move someone. The move can be the end at times and I am greatly aware of this for Mom.

I continue to bring her her favorite foods, which include bananas, a Snickers bar, salted peanuts, a burger with fried onions, or a Dairy Queen Snickers Blizzard. Sometimes I find her just sitting at the table and her tablemate is gently reminding her to eat. I am grateful to her that she is looking out for Mom.

I try not to bring Mom to my home too much during this transition time because I want her to get used to her new life. But, every once in a while, I break her free and we head for a drive around my neighborhood and we end up at my home. The home that she has visited with my dad. The bedroom in our basement has always been hers, but I know she can't walk up and down those thirteen steps anymore, and the last time she stayed with me, she told me she was up all night and was voicing her confusion. She felt she had done something bad in the middle of the night and was worried about it. I never found out if she had broken something or was confused that it wasn't her own bed. But I know she carried it with her because she mentioned it a few times and it was something that she remembered. She kept telling me she didn't sleep the whole night and I believed her.

The rare days that I bring her to my home are filled by my girls. Normally we do some cooking or baking. I will always have wonderful memories of getting out her favorite cookbook, the *Fron Church Cookbook,* or simply called "The Book," and making her own recipes with my girls. I can tell she wants to track better and she studies the recipes. I watch her confusion appear. I make it into a game for my older daughter and we measure the ingredients together. Chili, lemon bars, rhubarb torte, and easy-bake cookies. Cooking and baking have always been in her life. Now that her life is slower, I want her to remain involved, even if I must help in the process. I can tell she wants to remember. She reads the recipes but just can't process what it all means. To watch this confusion with recipes is heartbreaking. I hate this disease.

After our time together ends, I bring her back to Clare Bridge. I usually park in the front of the building, grab her walker, and slowly get her out of my car. We walk through the front door and push the button that alerts them that we want to get in. My mom does not understand why we must do this and she asks me about it every single time. She tries to open the door and an odd-sounding noise shrieks loudly. I tell her we must wait for them to let us in and she continues to give me a blank look. Over the years, my girls will fight over who gets to push the button.

We slowly move down the hall and into her room. Every time we get to the door, she looks for the shadow box on the wall and there is her picture and all the people she loves placed with such love. We worked on the box together and she picked out the pictures she wanted in the box. There is a picture of her as a young woman. Another of her mother and her brothers and sisters. A picture of her cooking for the seniors in our hometown. Pictures of Ross, Sophia, Emme, and Mom and me. All the people who are important to her. We will look at this box more times than I can count. A simple box on a wall filled with memories.

On many occasions Mom's roommate is in the room and so is her daughter, who visits about the same amount as I do. The staff was correct in describing the daughter to me. Loud, opinionated, and at times obnoxious to the staff. She is a medical professional. She tells me immediately what she does for a living. She has started to rearrange my mom's items, pulling Mom's curtains shut when her own mom goes to bed. She has started to lecture me on what I should or should not bring for Mom. I have stocked Mom's room with her favorite treats: salted peanuts in a jar, mini Snickers in a bowl for staff, soft popcorn, and some bananas right by her bed. She critiques me on what I am buying for Mom. As you can imagine, I start to get annoyed. I am normally a person who doesn't like conflict. In fact, I hate conflict. Work, home, family. I can feel my pulse start to race and I just keep things inside until I start to cry. I'm not sure if that is normal, but that's how I handle it. This is another matter.

I start to visit when the woman is not there. I look up her work schedule online, since she told me where she works. But we still end up running into each other. I listen to her complain about how bad sweets are for the elderly and listen to her call my mom Jeannie. Over and over. It's Jeanne. Like bean. Clean. Dean. Queen. Like the Lemon Bar Queen that my friends and family call her. Each and every time I correct her. "It's not Jeannie, it's Jean with an extra n and an e." It's something Mom had not shared with many people, but I know it bothered her when people called her Jeannie. One woman in my hometown always called her Jeannie. One day we were walking past First National Bank and the woman shouted out hello. "Hi, Jeannnnnnie!" My mom under her breath said, "I hate when she calls me that." I have always remembered that and nicely correct people when they say her name incorrectly. She might not have liked the tone the woman used, but I will always remember that she whispered that, almost as a reflex.

I remind myself that if it gets too bad, I will talk to the office staff. I have a feeling they are aware of her many issues.

Mom and I are working on a puzzle this afternoon and she is very quiet. She turns to me and says, "Are you my pretty Jodi?" I remind her that I am and that she is my pretty mom. There is a long pause. She replies, "No, I am just pretty old." She continues to be my funny mom.

The Birthday, April 2013

My mom's birthday is tomorrow. She will be eighty-seven. When I think about that, I am amazed she has made it this far. She has lived a long and wonderful life. I reminded her yesterday that her birthday is Friday. She asked how old she would be and I said eighty-seven. "That can't be." Yes, Mom. "Boy, I'm old." Me, laughing.

When my dad died almost six years ago, I wasn't sure she would make it. It was difficult for her. He was the alpha male, the dominant one in the relationship. They had been married four days shy of sixty years. She was a good wife and they made it through some dark times. Many of those dark times revolved around his alcoholism and his quick temper and anger. But there was much love and a strong bond between the two of them. It is rare she doesn't talk about him in some context. "Boy, I miss Russ." I know he is watching over her and I hope he is happy with the way she is being taken care of. I miss his wisdom. There are days I wonder if I have made the right choices with her care. I wish heaven had a once-a-year call so you could just check in, see how things are going.

I know time with her is limited. I think of that when she's not having a good day. I try remembering her past birthdays and how she never wanted gifts but just wanted to be together. Family is important in times like this. I am the same age today as my mom was when she adopted me. Forty-three. I also remember how important birthdays were to Mom and how she celebrated ours with joy. We were a gift to her. One that she and my dad wanted for a very long time. She really has it turned around. She is our gift and has touched and blessed many lives.

I asked what she wanted for her birthday. She'd like to see me and eat Chinese food. I think I can handle that.

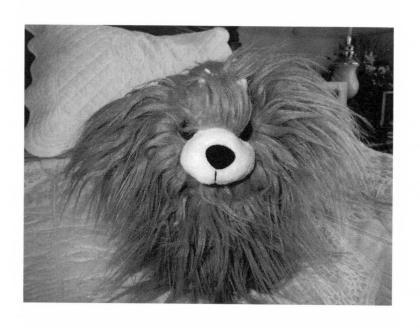

Matilda

"Have you met my dog?" This happens every day I visit. Our conversation is on repeat. I think it's funny she calls it Matilda. That was the name she called me when I was younger and I knew I was in trouble. "You'd better clean that room, Matilda" or "Listen, Matilda."

This dog came out of nowhere and ended up on Mom's bed one afternoon. I brought it to the nurses. They looked at the tag, which had another woman's name written on it. She had passed away last month. They said if Mom wanted to keep her, she could. How do they know it's a her?

I brought her back to Mom's room and she seemed angry I took her in the first place. This is Mom's dog. It is hairy and I had to bring some Febreze to eliminate odor. I'm not sure where it's been, but I'm stuck sharing Mom with Matilda.

She's never been a huge dog lover. Dad and Ross had hunting dogs so she didn't get a choice really. Our one dog that she was close to was named Rusty. Maybe a little similar to Matilda.

On the positive side, Matilda has brought her such joy. She takes her everywhere. She's traveled quite a bit in the last few months. We brought her to Ruby Tuesday, the doctor's office (where the doctor let Mom hold her during her chest X-ray), the eye doctor, Easter brunch, and on a car ride where she kept showing the dog to people who had stopped by us at a light. I'm sure they thought we were nuts. Mom would hold her so she'd be looking out the window. All the residents know it is Mom's and ask to pet it. Some days I'm not sure if she knows it's fake. She has started talking to it a lot. Now I find myself talking to Matilda. Great.

On the flip side, she pays more attention to the dog than to me, and I have to keep track of it when we go out. I am now all right with that. I have to be. It has brought her smile back, which had been lost in the last year with her disease. On occasion my girls would get a smile out of her. But it was rare. I missed that smile. Matilda has brought it back. For that, I am thankful.

The Voice

In 1990, I started my first week of nursing assistant classes. I had discovered that my first rotation would be at a nursing home in downtown Minneapolis. I remember feeling fearful and worried because I didn't know where it was or what to expect. I called my dad, who told me to take a trial run first and that I would be just fine. I did take a trial run and remember getting all turned around. One-way streets, police everywhere, no idea where to park. I'm grateful I listened to my dad or I would have been lost on my very first day.

I remember my first day there like it was yesterday. The long hallway leading to the Alzheimer's Unit. To unlock the door, I had to input the year using the keypad. I was so nervous being in this unit. As we were being assigned our first patients, I hoped mine would be not a man but a gentle female. Ann, my teacher stated, was picked just for me.

I remember reading her chart and her history. The first word was simply *DEMENTIA*. Information about her family and a short health history were listed. I thought to myself, I can handle this.

I gathered my paperwork and went to find her room. I knocked on her door. Ann was sitting in her wheelchair, wide awake. She gave me a half smile. I introduced myself and started asking her questions. I'm sure I overwhelmed her with my eagerness. As I look back, I was naïve. I kept asking her questions but was not getting a response. I reworded questions and statements and still she did not speak. I didn't know what to do. Did I miss something in her chart? Why is she not telling me her name? Why is she ignoring me and just giving me a sweet, shy smile?

I excused myself and went to find my teacher. I explained the problem to her. My teacher told me that at the end of the month, I need to give a report on her as a case study. Great, I thought.

So for the next month Ann and I met every day. I would go home at night, consult my nursing books, and think of ways I could get her to speak. I hated that this disease had robbed her of her voice. Every day I would take her out of her room, where she preferred to stay, and bring her to a different destination. We found the huge windows that faced the freeway, Highway 94. We strolled the hallways and watched all the people waiting to catch the bus. We attended activities in the building. I noted that she loved to hear people sing. I even caught her humming. But no words ever escaped her lips. For one month I tried my best to get her to speak. Time was running out; I had only a week left with her.

I attended to her needs, gave her medication and sat with her. I'm sure she got sick of me telling her about my day, how nervous I was to drive in this area, and my goal to become a registered nurse one day.

During that month, I never saw a family member come to visit her, and it made me angry. She was never a behavior problem. She never shouted out or grabbed somebody. Why wouldn't someone come and see this lovely woman?

I loved seeing her. This woman, even without words, made my day. On my last day with her, we sat by the big window on the floor, sun streaming through, and watched the people walk by. I told her it was my last day at the nursing home but if I was able, I would come see her again.

I glanced at her and saw tears slowly streaming down her face. She reached over and patted my hand. I can still picture her small veined hand on my own nineteen-year-old hand. She finally communicated with me and I struggled not to cry. After that whole month of trying my hardest, I finally got more than I needed from her.

It has been twenty-four years since I saw Ann. She is long gone, but she has stayed with me.

I thought of Ann when my cousin Bart called to say he wanted to bring his dad, my mom's brother, to visit her tomorrow. I was so happy to hear this. Not many people visit Mom. I told him the visit may not last long but that I was so happy to hear he wanted to see her.

Family is important, even if you can't communicate. Who knows how long Ann's voice had been missing? Maybe her family just didn't want to come or it was too hard for them. Even without a voice, these patients welcome visitors. Just so we are clear, Mom still has her voice. Boy, does she ever. I love to hear her talk about the birds, ask me where Matilda, her dog, is, and voice her concerns that I need to get home because it's snowing.

Sometimes sitting with loved ones is all they need. You will never know how much it will touch them or touch you.

The Displacement, May 2013

I got home and looked up the word *displacement* today. It's a term I have been struggling with quite a bit. I want to make sure it accurately describes how I feel on occasion. I was right. In simple terms, displacement is when we have a bad day at work and come home crabby and irritable and yell at the dog, the kids, and anyone in our way. Are you really mad at them or is it the effects of your bad day? Have you taken your anger out on them?

I could give you fifty examples of displacement with the families I have dealt with. They are mad that their loved one is ill. The patient finds out bad test results or they know they don't have much time left. They are mad and you are there. It's not a daily occurrence, but it happens enough that I should know what it is and when it comes along.

A year ago I took care of a woman with a daughter who lived out of town. She sent me critical emails about her mom's care and what we were doing wrong. I would see her email in my inbox and my heart rate would accelerate. I did not want to open them. There was no pleasing this family. Their mother was having a difficult time with her memory loss. She was a woman in her early sixties and the children were having a difficult time with the diagnosis. I could relate. Their anger was normally directed at our staff and me. We were the ones in charge. I know it was not about me, but rather their grief; I was just in their direct line of fire.

Displacement. I think I have it. I am still having a tough time with my mom's roommate's daughter. I know how stressful it is to lose your mom to this disease. Her mom cannot communicate and she is very different than my mom. I think how hard this must be for this daughter.

But still.

She continues to rearrange my mom's stuff, lectures me on the number of mini-Snickers bars I buy for her, still calls my mom by the wrong name, and will let me know that Mom is not brushing her teeth enough.

It's been a while since I've met such a woman. I feel sometimes that the air is being sucked out of me when she is in the room. She takes up the whole space. I breathe differently every time she is there.

She continues to tell me that she is a medical professional, just like me but at a much higher level. She has told me 500 times what she does. I learned that the daughter talked to a social worker friend of mine, who was in her office for a medical visit. The daughter told my friend how appalled she was at how much candy the daughter of her mother's roommate gave her, among other things. My heart broke. I realize what a small world we live in. The social worker friend and I connected that the daughter was actually talking about my mom and me in her words of shame. After a few months, I gathered the courage to confront her. It did not go well. I asked her to please not talk about my mom. Now she ignores me and has reported me to the building administrator. Their office has been very understanding.

When I think of how I should have handled this in a different way, I am reminded of displacement. Am I displacing my anger on the daughter because of my loss of Mom? Should I have kept my feelings to myself? Why does this woman bother me so much? Does she think I am a bad daughter because I give Mom candy? Questions I am not sure of. We are both dealing with grief. Maybe our grief is one and the same, but we are handling it in a different way. Loss is loss no matter how you look at it.

For the record, I am still buying Mom nuts and Snickers. If she only has one month left on this planet, I hope she goes down with a Snickers bar and coffee in her cup right beside her. As it should be.

I think if you can understand displacement and what it means, that is the first step. Baby steps for me and a few glasses of wine this week.

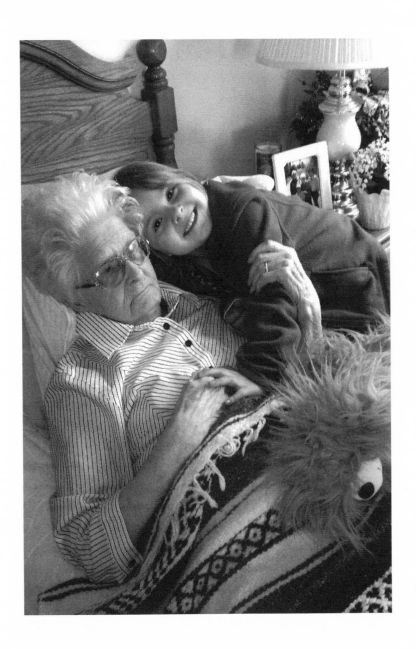

Touch

Last week I took the picture on the previous page. It was one of those special days where we stopped by on a whim. Emme wanted Jimmy John's for lunch and we brought Mom a loaded ham sandwich. Since I moved her into Clare Bridge, she hasn't been eating as much, which has worried me. I've been bringing her some of her favorite treats, but I notice she hasn't been eating them. She was excited to see that the ham sandwich had tomato on it and she ate half of it, along with those salty, crispy chips. It was such a good thing to watch her eat.

We walked back to her room and my mom and Emme both headed for the bed. They watched a game show. The picture shows Mom watching TV and Emme, as normal, snuggling with her grandma. I love how they touch each other. They seem to have a quiet communication. I think the picture captures both of them so well.

I was thinking today of how important touch is. There are many statistics regarding touch, including increased blood flow and nerves firing. A few months ago I had a conversation with one of my long-term clients. I have taken care of her for close to nine years. She told me that the only time she gets any kind of physical contact is when I hug her on my nursing visits. That was an eye-opening comment for me. By nature, I am not really a hugger. I will hug someone if I feel that comfort level with them. Some people, I have learned, don't like to be touched or hugged. I am careful of that with nursing.

The previous weekend I opened a hospice case for a man who broke his hip and femur. The family decided not to put him through surgery since he would most likely not have survived. I found him in bed, wearing his World War II hat, in so much pain. He had all of his family around, including his sweet wife. She was in a memory care unit and she was thinking he was her father. It was a difficult moment. I sat by his bed and he whispered something to me and touched my face. I could not really hear what he said, but the daughter behind me started to cry. She felt that he thought I was his wife. So gentle and sweet. Those are the times that mean so much. I saw him yesterday for my visit and sat with him. His breathing was now labored and I'm sure it will be his last day. We talked about his family and his wife, and I held his hand. I know he knew both the home health aide and I were there. Big-band music was playing in the background. His favorite hat was in place. Again, thinking of how important touch is.

Remember that when you reach out to someone, if only for a quick hug or touch on the arm, it does mean something.

Mother's Day

Tomorrow is Mother's Day. I think we should honor our mothers every day. In my card to Mom, I gave her some reasons why I love her.

1. She could make anyone fall in love with rhubarb. Really. Jam, torte, sauce, pie, bars, and bread. Her love of rhubarb and baking with it was well known. I almost called my blog The Rhubarb Queen.

2. She would send me stamps throughout college. I know what her thinking was behind that. Pay bills and send letters to Mom. I was on to her but, boy, did I love getting those stamps in the mail. Something I will carry on with my girls.

3. She taught me that life is hard work. And she has a bad back to show it. She never sat still long unless she was reading. I love that about her.

4. She stressed the importance of reading. She would tell me, "When you don't know what to do or if you are sad, get a good book." I can't tell you the amount of time I spent with her on their big bed, both of us reading a book. If I could capture that moment in time, I would hang it on my wall.

5. Marriage is hard, but stick with it. She and my dad found their way to sixty years. She deserves a medal. Well, maybe a statue.

6. She taught me that clothes are best hung on the line. During the summer, we rarely used the dryer, and there is no smell on earth like sheets taken off the line.

7. You are never too old to try something. Mom's favorite game was Scrabble. She took the game VERY seriously. Ask my family. A few months ago, I showed her Words With Friends on my iPad. It took her a few times but she got the concept and could think of some words to play. WWF players, you may be playing my mom.

8. Keep your friends close. Mom has been lucky. She has wonderful friends who still look out for her. I know she can feel that. Friends are a blessing and she has been truly blessed.

9. She could spend the whole day ironing. She tried to impress the fact that crisp shirts, pants, and sheets look sharp. I am still working on this and I know she would be shaking her head right now if she saw my work pants.

10. Try your best to be a good mom. In the past, she talked about some issues she felt she didn't handle the best she could. Trivial things that I would hardly blink an eye at, but to her they meant something. I try. Some days I knock it out of the park. Other days I feel I am the worst mom and daughter. She was long ago forgiven. I hope I turn out as well as my mom.

Bingo

I played a little Bingo with Mom today. It's something I do with her only a few times a month. When you mention the word *Bingo* to my Mom, her ears perk up and she wants to know what time the game starts. No other phrase excites her more except when we talk about her grandchildren.

I walk with her down the long hallway and prepare myself for the chaos. If you have never been to Bingo at a memory care unit, you may have difficulty picturing it, but I'll try to explain.

People just love to play Bingo. Everyone comes out of their room and tries to get the "best" cards, which I think is so funny. Many people also play three cards at once. Yes, memory care residents playing three cards at once.

In the first thirty minutes there will be ten false alarms for Bingo. No, make that twenty. The person who calls the numbers has the patience of Mother Teresa. I am currently on my third cup of coffee trying to channel calmness and serenity while listening to the false alarms. I now know I can't come after work when I'm tired. "B-4." "What was that? Can you call it again? What did the woman say? B-5?"

Emme was slapped on the hand once for playing with the cards next to one woman. Emme is only four, and we had to move since the woman was playing "for keeps." I have learned that the woman is just fine one-on-one. Just don't sit by her at Bingo.

People love the $1 prizes, when they actually win. Mom won a photo holder and she liked it better than any other gift I have given her. "Can you believe I won this frame?"

When I watch Mom play Bingo, I see how focused she is on her game. It's amazing to watch. She doesn't remember what she had for lunch or what day it is. Some days she cannot even recognize my face or name. But she can concentrate on Bingo. She can tune the other players out and focus on her game. The brain is an amazing organ that receives and interprets data. I wish I could get in that control center and tinker around. Fix what needs to be fixed. Return her to her days of baking, reading, driving, and helping others.

She has won some cheese and crackers this afternoon and she is happy. She has her coffee, crackers, Bingo, her stuffed dog Matilda, and me.

The Catacombs

Somewhere in the catacombs of my mom's brain, the memory and history of me has been tucked away. One of the hardest things I have struggled with is my mom not remembering who I am. How could she forget my face, my voice, my job as a nurse, or even Sophia's name?

I remember the first time she forgot. It is etched in my own brain. We were playing Bingo about six months ago and she turned to me and quietly asked if I was "her Jodi." I reminded her that I was and always would be her Jodi. I realize I should not have been surprised. But I was. Very surprised and deeply sad.

Not long ago I had a conversation with Mom's neurologist, whom I adore. She is gentle, mild-mannered, wicked smart, and someone who does not mind my endless questions. We connect and she connects with Mom. She reminded me that Mom may not remember or recognize me at forty-three. She may picture me at the age of seventeen or even thirty. She may not remember that I have grown to be an actual adult. I am hoping she remembers me at twenty-seven, fresh out of nursing school and having just met Steve, my husband. That was a good year.

On Mother's Day this year, she sat in my big chair in our sunroom and looked at me and asked, "Where is Jodi?" The doctor's words of wisdom popped in my head. I told her it was me and she nodded.

I know the first time she did it she was sad. I could feel her deflate and get quiet. I am sure she was also thinking the same thought. How could I forget her? I know in my heart there will be a day where she will totally forget me. I am heartbroken at the thought. But what you do today matters. We read mail together, play Bingo, watch old shows, and go for slow walks. I know in the catacombs of cells and matter of her brain, I will always take up space. The space, I imagine, gets smaller every day. But it will always be there. Never really going way.

Laughter

This week, I choose to laugh. I think when you watch a loved one disappear every day you can decide that you will be sad, fearful, overwhelmed, or depressed. I am all of these at times. But a laugh will awaken your senses, bring things back in perspective, and get you back on track. This is what made me laugh in the past week.

We found my mom's remote for her TV. We bought her this great new TV when she moved in and within ten days she lost the remote. I have looked high and low for this remote. In a memory care unit, things disappear. I understand this. Almost every day I searched and checked with the nursing staff, finally giving up and just keeping her favorite channel on WCCO.

Last week, her phone rang when I was there and she used the remote to answer. I looked at her table and saw that next to the phone sat the remote, as if it had been there the whole time. After six months and all that searching, it had mysteriously showed up. For months now, Mom's alarm clock has been on the floor. I keep thinking she has been messing with it and just doesn't pick it up or that she is tripping over the cord. When I called last week, she said there was a man in her room and they were talking. She didn't seem annoyed by it, but I called the front desk and they got him out. That was my first clue. When I went last week, Mom and I were lying on her bed watching a Western on TV and the man walked straight into her room, totally oblivious to us lying there. He went around the bed and proceeded to unplug her clock, shuffle past us, and walk out of the room with it. I watched with amusement the culprit who was the Clock Stealer. Mystery solved. He was very sweet, and when I spoke to the nurses, I learned he used to be an engineer, just like my dad. I think he was very interested in her clock. Now I see he is in her room all the time. I see him holding his clock, walking down the hallway. I think Mom may have liked his company.

When I went to visit Mom last week, I met her in the beauty shop. There she was happily getting her hair done. When I looked to Mom's right, there was a woman looking closely at her. She had Mom's sweater on. Then I looked closer and saw she also had her pants and even her shoes on. The beauty shop assistant and I had a giggle. You know this happens in a memory care unit. It is a small event that left us all with a good laugh. She even looked like Mom.

In the scope of my mom's life, things will, at times, make me mad. But it's important for me to laugh. The staff work so hard at making sure things are correct. I will say it again: They have an awfully tough job. Some are spit on, pushed, screamed at, called vulgar names, and not given the respect they deserve. I remember my first nursing assistant job like it was yesterday. Four years in a memory care unit. Patience and laughter are key. Kindness to the staff goes a long way.

The Devotional, June 2013

Today I got to spend some time with Mom. We have hired a wonderful college student, Rachel, for the summer to watch the girls. I now get to spend Wednesday mornings with Mom without the girls. It's a nice break for me and it's much quieter. I don't want it to be a chore for the girls to come. I want them to *want* to see Grandma on their own terms. I am happy they still want to see her. For children so young, they understand her loss some days better than I do.

Today, I caught Mom sleeping in the chair. She has been sleeping more often. I know that for eighty-seven years old, she does pretty well physically. I brought her some magazines and her Matilda was huddled next to her. That crazy, ugly dog.

I last saw her on Sunday. We talked about the next book I would read to her. There are many things my mom has forgotten. I could not begin to count the number of hours we have read together. I would read a great book and send it to Starbuck and she would read it in days. She has always had a little more time than I to read. We would discuss what we loved or hated about it and she would ask for more. Many of my special books in my library are from her. A sweet reminder of the love we have shared.

Today, I told her about the book I have been reading, *Orphan Train*. She was interested in the topic and I told her we could read it after I am finished. We picked up her devotional book and I was about to read her the June 12 devotion when I asked her if she would read it to me. She had last read on Sunday and it was a joy to hear her voice again. Time escaped back to the days of hearing her read scripture for church, reading her Bible, reading stories to the girls, and reading recipes she loved. She had a strong yet sweet rhythm to her reading. I miss that voice. I told friends that for months I have been reading to her. But she fooled me just a little. There were times when she would fall asleep while I was reading to her and I would watch her nap and then I'd quietly leave. Reading to her was just as much enjoyment for me as it was for her. I wish that whatever causes this damn disease would leave that part of her brain alone.

This is what Mom read to me today. It's a wonderful passage.

"Let me help you get through this day. There are many possible paths to travel between getting up in the morning and lying down at night. Stay alert to the many choice-points along the way, being continually aware of my presence. You will get through this day one way or the other. One way is to moan and groan, stumbling alone with shuffling feet. This will get you to the end of the day eventually. But there is a better way. You can choose to walk with me along the path of peace, leaning on me as much as you need. There will be difficulties along the way, but you can face them confidently in my strength."

Hearing her voice again was magical.

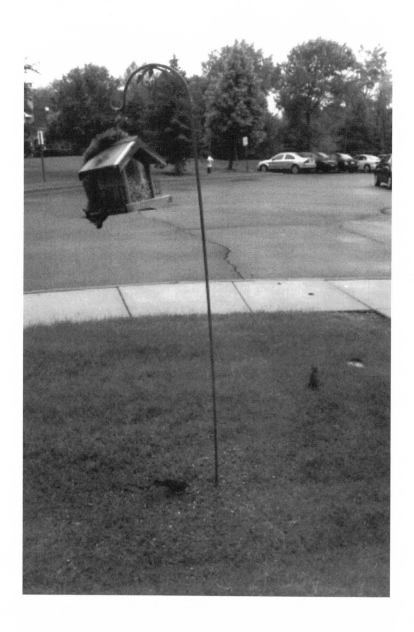

The Lie

Over the past week, my mom's eyes have been glued to the bird-house outside her roommate's window. She can sit in her chair, look to her right, and watch all the excitement that goes on all day long. Today, there has been a lot of action.

Today, we spent an hour watching the crazy behavior of the bunnies, the birds, and a squirrel trying to chase one another and get at the bird feeder. My mom's enjoyment was contagious. She then told me the same thing she has been telling me for one solid week. "You know, I made that birdhouse." Every time I'm here she tells me about the birdhouse and how proud she is of it.

At first, I went along. She was matter-of-fact, bold, and very direct. You are taught as a nurse to go along with a person with memory loss, unless their statement will hurt them. You try to reduce their anxiety. I have heard so many stories over the years. An eighty-year-old woman stating her mother was here with her or a man telling me that we had just been on a cruise together. You know their comment is untrue. But if I said to the woman, "Your mom died fifty years ago," or "You and I have never been on a cruise together," you will add to their confusion, make them feel unworthy, and increase their anxiety. Sometimes it depends on the situation, but I normally just go with the flow.

At first, I asked the nursing staff if she really did make the birdhouse. I didn't want to assume that she hadn't. They reported she had not made it. Mom even told Steve on Father's Day that she had made this wonderful birdhouse. When she told me again and I said I had heard about it, she answered with disappointment, "You don't think I made it." It was the look she gave me. Sad, quiet, with remorse. My tone must have alerted her that I didn't believe her. She looked away and was quiet. I told her, "Mom, if you tell me that you made it, I believe you." I was disappointed in myself that I didn't come across better toward her and I know she must have felt that.

A few months ago, she asked me how much her rent was. In the last few years, she has not asked me one question about bills, her checkbook, rent, hair, medication expense, or how I pay for her things. She has forgotten that piece of her life. Again, I was not as truthful as I should have been. If she knew what the cost was, it would upset her. I kept it in the ballpark, but a few thousand dollars less. Does she really need to know the cost? Yes, if I was being honest. Would it add to her anxiety and worry? Yes, for sure. Would I lie again so she would not worry? Yes, I would lie again so she would not worry.

I'm looking at the birdhouse and thinking to myself, I have spent the last hour watching this with Mom. My own bills to pay, family activities to think about, work always on my mind, and things I have put off. This time with her is important. Yes. She did make that birdhouse, just so we are clear.

The Walk, July 2013

Walking my mom back to her room tonight, I am reminded how much she has slowed down. She left her walker back in her room, so I go get it and return to walk her again. I know tonight is not the best night to go for a walk. She is tired, so very tired. I can see it in her face and even in the way she tries to get up. She bends her knees, grabs for the table, and tries to pull herself up. She is worried about her coffee and I am worried about how I'm going to get her back to her room.

For those of you who don't know, my mom has always been a walker. Walking has given her pleasure, kept her slim and trim, and given her much time for her thoughts. When I was in college, I would call for Mom, and Dad would say, "She walked to the Dairy Queen," or "She walked to get the mail and stop by Pete's." She would walk in my hometown, and when they wintered in Yuma, she picked a route close to their home. My dad told me that once she passed a house to talk to some children in the yard and a pit bull chased her. She was not walking in the best neighborhood, and both my dad and I encouraged her to change her route.

After I graduated from high school I would come home for a visit and we would always go for a walk. It was a time to catch up, talk about nursing school, boys, books that we were reading, and my brother. She was a fast walker, and so was I. We always ended up at the DQ and talking with her friends.

When Mom started to get confused, friends would call me and say she kept getting turned around. She would ask people how to get back home. I think I was in a little bit of denial. After all these years and all of her walks, how could she forget her way home? One of the hardest calls was from one of her friends, stating that Mom got confused coming home from the grocery store. The store is only two long blocks away. She had asked a stranger where her house was. In a small town, the story came back to me. My heart was sad. One of the things I did not want her to give up was her nightly walks. Could she walk with friends? Maybe she could just walk in the daytime?

Soon after that, we moved her to Holly Ridge. She walked to church a few times, but the staff and I were worried about her not getting back. "I can walk to church; it's only a few blocks away." Saying no to her was hard. You find yourself saying no to so many things that mean so much to her.

Fast-forward a few years now and we are still walking: slow, steady, but nowhere near what I remember. As I watch her now, I see her left foot is dragging a little, her back is bent with osteoporosis, her hands are gripping the walker, and her breathing is labored. Tired.

I'm sure a wheelchair will be the next step. But I can barely get that word out of my mouth. I am praying she will keep those legs moving for a while, just like she has done for the last eighty-seven years. Tomorrow I'm going to take her outside if it's nice. We're going to check "her" bird feeder. Tomorrow is a new day.

The Light

I haven't felt like writing much lately, which is unusual. Normally I journal ideas in my beautiful leather-bound book my sister-in-law Wendy gave me. But we have been busy with vacation, baseball, Emme's fifth birthday, my work, and a few 5K races. My biggest concern is that Mom has been sick since we got back.

I noticed it during my first visit after our trip. I found her lethargic, running a temp, barely able to keep her head up, and in a wheelchair. I had never witnessed her so ill. As a nurse, I had all of the symptoms running through my mind. Stroke, too much Ultram for pain, heart ... you get the picture. She even refused her beloved coffee, so I knew that she was very ill.

For some time I have noticed Mom's inner light and brightness dimming. Her list of accomplishments is amazing and I won't bore you with everything she has brought to this world. Those of you who know her understand how much she has meant to so many. To watch her decline and lose that inner light is tough. I see it in patients I take care of. They say, "I'm tired," and I know what they mean. They battle cancer, Parkinson's, stroke, heart issues, dementia. They know and I know. Life gives us a set number of years; what we do with that is up to us. End-of-life issues are tough on everyone, and I am always understanding when someone says they are ready.

Mortality sets in. Many of Mom's friends have died, she's away from her hometown that she loved, and she doesn't get many visitors. My brother hasn't seen her since last November. She can't cook, read, get the mail, drive a car, call me on the phone, or even pay a bill. I think that my light would also dim. She has lived a long life and I am mindful of that. Yes, we want our loved ones to live on, but I understand how tired they can get. They are ready for it to be over. Mom is tired, but I believe she has accomplished everything she set out to do. She is ready, be it today, next week, or a year from now.

I am thankful for all the staff who take such good care of Mom. Even her wonderful beautician asked about her. That means a lot.

This morning's conversation after I find out she is feeling better:

Mom: Who brought me bananas?
Me: I did. I know that you love them.
Mom: How do you know that?
Me: I know what you like, so I buy them for you.
Mom: Well, if you knew what I liked, you would bring me Snickers instead of bananas.

Point well taken.

The Visitor, August 2013

Years ago, when I first became a nursing assistant, I worked in an Alzheimer's unit for four years. It was a place that I loved, and I learned a lot about life and nursing. I had to become good at bribes, distraction, negotiation, breakdowns, agitation, sadness, and grief. Every day was different and I learned to adapt pretty quickly. The unit also taught me about love, family, hope, and the effort families would go through visiting their loved ones. I remember one woman who would visit her husband every single day, without fail. Even with his end-stage dementia, she could still bring a smile to his face.

My favorite residents were the ones who did not have any family visit them. Even though it has been almost twenty years, I can still picture them and their names. Ethel, who always had perfect hair and a slight drool, would ask me if I had seen her mother today. John, who had had a stroke and would allow only me to get him dressed and would never hit me, like he would the other staff. If I didn't have him on my schedule, I would trade him for another resident. He couldn't communicate, but every time he would see me, he would start to cry. I adored him and no one could understand why since he was so combative. There was Helene, who was aggressive and hit me in the head so hard one day I saw my first stars. We became friends after that and when she was having a very bad day we would talk about her family and she would slowly start to calm down. I know that it was the disease and that she didn't mean to hurt me.

I miss those days of one-to-one care. I believe those four years were the best thing that could have happened to me and made me want to continue my nursing education. It has helped me under-stand this disease and has prepared me for my journey with Mom.

When you have a loved one who is battling a disease, whether it be Alzheimer's, Parkinson's, cancer, or stroke, it can be hard to visit them. The unknown is a powerful thing. Your friend or loved one may look different, act strangely, move in a way you are not used to, or forget who you are. You need to prepare yourself for that. My brother has not visited my mom for a while. I am not going to fault him for that. I know that when you hear a diagno-sis of a disease, fear can overtake you. It can be difficult to watch your loved one change. I think that this has been hard for him. I reminded him not long ago that she is still in there. She still looks the same but may not remember your name. She is still our beau-tiful, funny, coffee-loving mother.

He came to see her last Saturday, a beautiful, perfect day. He and his girlfriend, Heather, arrived and I prepped Mom by stat-ing his name, in case she forgot. He was nervous. I showed him around, introduced him to the staff and her stuffed dog, Matilda. We also spent some time outside, which Mom enjoyed. I haven't asked him to do much with her care, though any help is appreci-ated. The hard part of my being a nurse is that he just lets me make the hard choices with her. His unspoken job is to call her. I will keep paying the expense of her phone so they can communicate on his terms.

At times, this is difficult for me. For twenty-plus years, I watch families and friends not visit. I have heard all the excuses and at times I want to shout at them. Even if you stay for five minutes or one hour or the whole day, it helps. For that amount of time, you have shown them you care. Even if they don't know who you are, I believe they feel your love and attention for that very moment. For that moment in time for them, you are in their world, you are present for them, and you make them feel worthy. And that is really what it's all about.

The Pity Party, September 2013

I'm having a pity party. Just a party of one today. I am thinking about some issues I have been working on in my brain and needing my mom to help me get through it.

We all have people in our lives who are our go-to people. They know our secrets, know how our brain works, and would never judge us on our choices. We talk to that special person about things that matter to us. That person is my mom.

Over the years, this has changed, as you can imagine. I am watchful and careful about the things I tell her. Many times she will remember only snippets of our conversation. Or she will remember some of it and be worried. She doesn't know this but I have kept certain issues private, not really sure how much she will understand and wanting to save her the worry if she does remember.

There are many reasons to hate this disease but one of the top reasons is that it has robbed my mom's brain of all the years of memories. I was trying to explain this to a girlfriend a while ago. The best way to describe it is that her brain is like a community filled with memories. So much is kept in that small community. Memories like getting us ready for the school year, working at Lutheran Social Services and cooking for the seniors, singing in the choir, attending my sporting events, working in her garden, walking, and enjoying her friends. All of that is kept up in that small community of her brain. But there is a wicked storm that is invading her community/brain and it's called Alzheimer's disease. It's a storm that nobody wants to see and it has caused destruction and sadness. It has damaged her community.

Over the years, she has guided and listened to me on so many issues and struggles, always with a suggestion, a solution, or just a simple comment like "I know you will get through this." I don't have that anymore and I miss it.

Ambiguous loss is a difficult road. She is physically there, yet in such a different context. It's a roller-coaster ride that we are both on and really would like to get off because it is making us both ill.

So for today, just attend my pity party. I'll get through this day and know that tomorrow it will be better. I'm off to see Mom and hopefully play some Bingo.

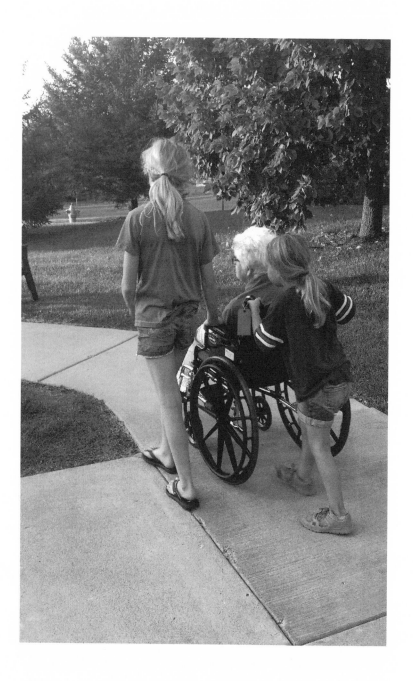

The Granddaughter

Yesterday I got to capture the sweetest moment with my mom and Sophia, my soon-to-be ten-year-old. If it's a day that I've been unable to see Mom, I try to call her before she goes to bed. It is a way that I connect with her and it usually gives me a laugh before bedtime. Her side of the conversation varies from suggestions to take her out for lunch or bring her more Snickers bars, to what she has done today. It is a short conversation but I enjoy it.

Sophia came in from outside and asked me if she could call Grandma tonight. I said, "All right, but remind her who you are right away so she doesn't hang up." She dialed the phone and went into her bedroom. I could hear her from the kitchen: "Hi, Grandma. It's Sophia. How are you?" Sophia proceeded to tell her about school, homework, biking to a friend's house, and her hockey practice. She asked what she had for dinner, whether she was in her jammies, and if she watched *Wheel of Fortune*. Just her tone in how she spoke to Mom made my heart ache with love. I wish I could have heard the other end of the conversation and how my mom answered her. It is by far the longest my mom has stayed on the phone. It might have been Sophia's gentle way, her not getting frustrated with her, and just agreeing with my mom. When their conversation was over, Sophia handed me the phone like it was no big deal. The first thing my mom said to me was, "I really enjoyed that." A few minutes later, I tracked Sophia down and told her how that made Grandma feel. Her response was "It was nothing." But it was something.

When I found out I was pregnant with Sophia, my parents were beyond thrilled. I think they might have been more excited than we were. My parents were seventy-seven at the time and had waited so long to be grandparents. The minute I told them, I know my mom started to make quilts. I could supply a small nation with the number of quilts she made for that baby. They waited patiently for nine months. I loved the attention, and my mom just thought of countless ways to love this baby.

When my water broke at midnight, we waited until the morning to tell them we were on our way to the hospital. They packed a bag and left Starbuck to drive two hours to Plymouth. I am sure my dad sped the whole way. Little did we all realize that Sophia had other ideas and she wasn't born until the following day at 3 a.m. My mom and dad stayed the whole time at the hospital and waited for their first grandchild to be born. When Steve finally came out to the waiting room, he said, "Oh boy, she's finally here." Of course, my dad heard *boy* first and was thrilled. I love that Steve had to tell him again, "It's a GIRL!" And so our love affair with her began.

If you could look in my mom's journals starting in 2003, you'd see that the entries are mainly about Sophia. I love how she wrote about her planned trips to come see her. They had a special kind of relationship, and I was so glad that they had that for almost five years, until Emme came along and there were two to love and, as you can imagine, Emme was just as loved. Both of the girls' middle names come from Mom's names. Sophia has spent ten years with Mom and has watched her memory fade. She is patient with her, even when she forgot about her last winter, which I know hurt her feelings. I reminded her that she would always be in Grandma's heart and that even if she couldn't get her name right, they had a close connection that would never go away.

I also reminded Sophia of all the trips we have taken with Grandma. For years, after my dad died, Sophia, Mom, and I traveled to some fun places. We spent time in Hayward, Bayfield, Madeline Island, Galena, Door County, and last year we took a trip to Wabasha, Red Wing, and Winona in southern Minnesota. The last trip was harder, so we ended our travels by taking the Padelford Riverboat tour up and down the Mississippi River with Captain Bob. We have gone for many car rides since. I am sad that our trips are over. We just need to make different memories.

To say I am proud of Sophia is an understatement. She has spent ten years with Mom and has gone through just as many high and lows. I hope she remembers all of this and keeps her heart open and can understand that none of us is perfect. To her, that conversation was no big deal. But to me, it was so much more.

The Hands, October 2013

When I called Mom last night, she said she had written a note for me but she couldn't find it. I could tell she was a little worried and it seemed important to her. I was happy yet surprised that she had put something down on paper. I do have her sign cards and she is always embarrassed her writing isn't what it used to be.

When I arrived today, she was getting her hair done. She was happy and funny and had forgotten about the note. I looked in her room and saw the note right by her chair. The paper was coffee stained (of course) and it read "My nails are in bad shape." Secretly, I was hoping for something else. Maybe "I love you" or "I need more Snickers." But I have to say the note made me smile. She had put something down and it made sense.

She had given me a note with her aging hands. Those beautiful hands that are now wrinkled, full of puffy veins, and with nails that need to be looked after. She was right. They do need attention.

Her hands have been busy for eighty-seven years: sewing beautiful, detailed quilts, changing my girls' diapers, or giving them a bath. She has held books in her hands and kept journals with details that she would eventually forget.

As I look at her hands, it seems like yesterday that I watched her canning corn and pickles. She loved to shuck the corn, gather the tomatoes or cucumbers, and fetch the water to boil. We loved the sound of the seal of the jar popping. She was so proud of being able to give her canned goods as gifts. She has cracked over a million eggs, kneaded bread from scratch, made her famous lemon bars, and squeezed doughnuts that melted in your mouth.

Her hands have sent me sweet, encouraging letters over the years, many times with stamps hidden in the letters. With those hands, she has kept a lovely garden, picked weeds and rocks in our farm fields, and gently fed a young calf. Her hands kept her busy as a farm wife, and I know she loved being on that farm while I was a child. Her hands have driven a car, mowed our lawn, signed many school papers, and swatted my bottom as a child. Now I watch her hold my girls, always touching them and loving them.

As I look over at them now, I see how much she has used them. Her wedding band still there after sixty-six years, shiny, well worn, and proof of her and my dad's love and devotion. She is proud of her ring, and at times I catch her playing with it, twisting and turning it around and around.

My sadness over what she cannot do anymore comes up from the bottom of my heart and spills out in tears as I write this. She may have forgotten all she has accomplished in her life but I haven't. She has used those hands to make a wonderful, busy life. When she holds my girls, I am reminded of this.

Her hands are not as busy as they used to be. But it's up to me to still hold them when I can. Today I get to hold her hands while she is getting her hair done. I have brought her a chocolate doughnut and we have coffee together. Even though I can't stay long with her today, I know she is having a good day. And, fittingly, they are going to can applesauce in the cooking area today. Perfect.

The Doctor's Visit, November 2013

1. When I decided to start writing a blog about Mom and our adventures, it was never my intention to be doom and gloom. The blog was just a glimmer of our life and the times we shared. Good times or not, we are a team and I have learned many things along the way. Some days I laugh. Some days I cry. Wednesday was her checkup with my doctor. I was excited for Mom to meet Dr. Woodland. I wanted her to get a flu shot. It was also a day for us to get out and have some fun. As I was thinking about how her day went, some things came to me that might help you if you take your loved one in for a doctor appointment.

2. Always know where the bathrooms are located. If you are confused as to why, you will soon find out.

3. If your loved one makes a comment about a man their same age being a "skeleton," it's okay to move over a chair or two. You might also want to tell them to use a quieter voice.

4. When checking your loved one's height, anticipate that they will argue over the shrinkage. "I'm not four-ten; I'm five-four." Maybe just let them think they are still five-four. (I knew she seemed shorter to me!)

5. The same applies to weight. (Mom has gained a few pounds but disagreed with our assessment that she had. I want her to gain some more weight but she is still in the mindset that "up a few pounds" is a tragedy.)

6. Never let them sit on the high examining table, even if they want to. (It almost gave me a heart attack getting her down.)

7. Assure them that the nurse is never trying to kill them when taking their blood or checking their blood pressure. I am a nurse and I know they really aren't trying to kill you.

8. When the doctor asks them what they did for a living and they look at you blankly and grab your hand, you may need someone to also hold onto your hand as well. (Sigh.)

9. If your loved one is like my mom, their labs may come back showing that their blood is 100 percent saturated with coffee.

10. It's always cold in the doctor's office. Bring a sweater or jacket—or try to turn up the heat on your own. Kidding!

11. When the doctor says to your loved one that it must be nice to be taken care of by your daughter and her response is "Which daughter?" knowing you are the only daughter, don't take it personally.

Overall, it was a good day and Mom checked out fine. I can hardly wait for the next appointment.

That Girl, December 2013

November was a long month for Mom and me. Not that anything really happened or that we ran into a problem. I guess I should say that it was long for me.

This month alone I worked on the following:

- Getting her a handicapped-accessible parking sticker. I'm not sure why I didn't think of it before. I can thank our wonderful doctor for reminding me that it's all right to get and use the sticker.

- I have been procrastinating working on her Medicare paperwork. To say it has been mind-boggling is an understatement.

- Every six months I have to prove to Social Security that her money is going to her care. I have to fill out another form with documented proof.

- I spent two hours with a Humana rep picking another plan for her because her original plan was discontinued. I will never get those two hours back.

- The Humana rep stated that she should have been taking advantage of a health and wellness plan where she gets free incontinence pads. Huh? He also stated that her dentist appointment in February should have been covered. Again, forms to fill out and hoping she gets $550 back.

- I spent two hours navigating the Humana site and signing her up for free supplies. Two hours.

- Paying bills, mailing Christmas cards, ordering pads, and keeping up with her medications and concerns that I have overall.

There are days I worry that I have no idea what I'm doing. As hard as I try, I worry about making a mistake that will affect her. What if I don't pick the right plan? Why didn't I understand that she would get free stuff every month? Why do I want to fall asleep watching this forty-five-minute video that Humana mandates I watch? I would do this for her a million times over but, at times, it is just plain hard. Very hard.

My birthday is November 7 and it was always a special day for my parents. When I was younger and we lived on the farm we had parties and invited all of our neighbors. Mom never missed calling me on my birthday or coming to see me. I think she loved the day more than I did.

On my birthday, I went to pick up some cupcakes for the nursing staff and to have coffee with Mom. She was in the entry-way and waved when she saw me through the door. She noticed the cupcakes and asked why I brought them. I did something that I rarely do with a person with memory loss. I asked her a question. "Mom, what's special about November 7?" We were walking slowly down the hallway and I could tell she was confused. "Is it an important day for me?" I tell her it's someone's birthday. Long pause. "I wish I could tell you." She doesn't remember. I know in my logical brain that I should not be sad. But for some reason, this year I was sad. November 7 did not ring a bell for her. I feel guilty for being sad.

We get to her room and we have coffee and cupcakes. I am lying on her bed and I catch her staring at me. I sometimes wonder if she really knows who I am. I can imagine in her brain that I am

"That Girl." That girl that brings her treats and bananas, makes her sign things she doesn't understand, tells her this is her home now and that I am her daughter. I am "That Girl" who walks with her, brings her grandchildren to see her, and watches the birds with her. I am not 100 percent sure she really knows it's me, Jodi.

When I came to see her a few days ago, I was talking to Mickey, the activity aide. She and I worked together twenty years ago at the nursing home. My mom, out of the blue, introduced me to Mickey and called me Jodi. Wow. For that moment, I was her daughter Jodi. I remember walking out of the building smiling.

The month has had ups and downs. There are some days when I can't make it over there because I'm tired. I know she is being taken care of well. But there is nothing like being there and checking on her. I call her at night and I can tell again when I am "That Girl." Her voice gets distant and she wants to get off the phone.

I miss the days when I was Jodi to her.

The Gladness and the Sadness, December 2013

Yesterday I found myself thinking about one of the families we take care of. This family has been difficult for me and I had an uncomfortable conversation with the daughter on Friday. As you can imagine with nursing, dysfunction is something that is a part of every case, to some extent. Part of your job is to remain neutral. Not judge. Just listen. Even if you feel their choices are not the choices you would make. Their issues have stayed with me because it is the holidays and their anger is palpable.

Loss and grief are hard, but when you add the holidays to the mix it can be incredibly difficult. In the last few weeks, we have lost five clients. Some were unexpected and some had been ill for a while. As you can imagine, their families are grieving. If loss were an object, it would be an ugly, prickly thing that never goes away. It's always present for some, from the time they get up in the morning to when they lay their head down at night.

It's hard getting to know them for a short period of time, seeing them at their worst, and then saying goodbye. It's always difficult for me to call the family to tell them how sorry we are. Grief and loss. Two difficult words. But with grief and loss come amazing stories. I'll share a few from the last few weeks.

One woman we took care of for a short while was a dancer, a theater lover, a painter, and a giving soul in our community. She declined quickly after losing her husband the previous year. Family surrounded her constantly; not one ounce of dysfunction in the family. It is rare that all family members are on the same page.

Her last days were filled with comfort, love, and a beautiful view of the river. Her son sang show tunes to her all night. He was close to her in bed and she quietly died lying next to him. What a beautiful way to go.

One client died a few weeks after that. She had a naughty cat that was, shall we say, misguided. I would tease her family and her caregiver, Roberta, that we needed to get rid of the cat. Her death was difficult for everyone. After she was gone, the cat sat on her empty hospital bed. Where is her owner? Is she coming back? Who can I scratch? Pets also feel loss.

A few days ago, a sweet, loving woman who was very ill told her daughter that her son was waiting in the living room for her but he had to go away for now and would be back tomorrow. The son she talked about had died years ago. She died the very next day. The story was a comfort for the family and I get goose bumps writing it.

So with their loss sometimes comes hope, love, and comfort. It's a hard time of year to lose someone. But just hearing their stories brings me a little comfort too. Ask any nurse and they will tell you that the holidays are a tough time of year.

With Mom, we go through the same thing. As in the last couple of years she and I have written a Christmas letter together and we have sent out forty cards. She has been receiving so many letters from friends and family and I've been hanging them up on her wall. The disease is a funny one. When I call her each night, she tells me that she received cards today. Every day is a new day and she forgets that the cards were sent in past days. In a way, I have to laugh. Every day she gets to start over and gets to enjoy her cards over and over again.

Christmas was an important time for her. When I saw her on Friday, she was worried about baking, buying the girls presents, and what she would make for the holiday. Every Christmas for my forty years, she cooked, baked, shopped, and wrapped gifts.

Her favorite things to make at Christmas were lefse, her famous cider, and her treats. I don't miss her Russian tea cake balls, which I teased her about being the worst cookies ever. She'd always put some in a box for me and I would give them away. There is gladness and sadness that she still gets to come to my house, even though she most likely will not remember it the next day.

Someone told me the other day that with grief, you can't ever fill that hole in your heart. But what you can do is cover your heart with love to protect that sacred hole. I agree.

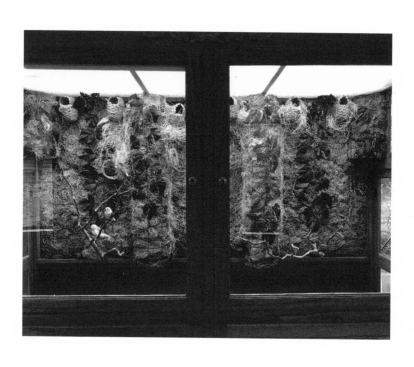

The Bag of Tricks, January 2014

Years ago, when I was a nursing assistant at North Ridge, I would walk a long hallway and go past a large structure filled with birds. There, watching quietly, would be many residents. On any given day they would be sitting there, ignoring people walking by to where they needed to go. They would find peace sitting there, just watching the birds flutter about and sing songs. I used to think it was sad, that their big enjoyment of the day was watching the birds fly around.

Fast-forward twenty years and I am now sitting here watching the birds with Mom. Today is a quiet day filled with busy people and residents walking around. There is an alcove where Mom and I sit in large wooden chairs, music quietly playing and the birds flying around. She is ignoring my questions and we sit here drinking coffee and I'm watching her as she watches the birds.

I find my mind wander a million miles away. I should be folding clothes, organizing our family calendar, paying bills. The girls are back in school after a long break and I haven't been to see Mom as often as I would like. Today, it's cold out and I feel the need to go. A girlfriend told me the other day, "Your mom won't know that you haven't been there in a while. She forgets." I know she is just being honest with me and I understand it. But *I* know if I haven't been there. My heart knows.

As I sit watching her, I think of how far we have come. Moving her closer to me, making all of her life choices. The hardness of it all. I was at the girls' hockey practice the other day and I was noticing all the grandparents watching their young players, clapping and cheering them on. It's so different for me. I wish she and my dad were here and able to watch the girls in their activities, cheering them on and being proud of them. My dad would have loved to see Sophia skate.

As we watch the birds, I think of a few days ago when I got the call from her memory care unit telling me she was refusing to get up. She was dressed but simply wanted to stay in bed. I got to leave work a little early and I stopped by Lunds grocery store and got her some peach pie and bananas. I arrived in her room and showed her what I purchased. She was less than interested and was irritable with me. Something was different about today and I thought of my nursing bag of tricks to get her up. Coffee. Pie. Matilda. Nothing worked and I was all right with her staying in bed. She's soon to be eighty-eight; she's earned her right to stay in bed. But what worked were those crazy birds. "Let's go see the birds, Mom!" She gave me a direct look, and said, "All right, let's go!"

Those bright, colorful, noisy, crazy birds make her content. So I'm content. The need to do everything today has passed for a moment and I'm spending time with her. I know the days with her are numbered and it's like a large clock ticking away. If every day I spend with her is watching the birds, that's fine. Maybe this is a way for me to slow down and relax too. I'm adding that to my bag of tricks.

The Boring Topic, February 2014

Today I am writing with Mom. Just so we are clear, she knows that I write about her. She feels that she is a terrible topic and she wonders why anyone would find her interesting. I reminded her also that I write about her because it was a suggestion of the Alzheimer's Association and that some of the issues we run into may help other people. She continues to think that she is a boring topic.

We have just finished lunch, and Bingo will start soon. We are reviewing our week. It goes something like this:

- We have lost her remote . . . we have found her remote. We have lost her remote . . . we have found her remote. Repeat times ten.

- She has found a new friend, a soft blue stuffed dog. She has not named it yet and I can tell that she has forgotten about Matilda for now. Matilda is sitting on top of her bed, watching the new dog taking her place. I hope we don't have to bring both of them on our travels. I hope future visitors bring food, not more stuffed animals. We decided to call her new dog Blue Dog. I know, creative.

- She has wanted to go home for the last month, and today is no different. I don't know where she thinks "home" is. She normally will tell me she wants to go home on the phone. Home could be one of a few places. It could be the farm we lived on for seventeen years with her lovely garden. It could be two blocks from my own house, where they lived when they adopted both Ross and me. It could be off of Chicago or Penn, where they lived in the forties and fifties. Home could be Howard Lake, where she graduated from and where she has so many memories. She also talks a lot about the red house, located in Crystal, where they lived for a short time. Home is important to people, and when illness occurs I hear that so much. "I want to go home!" When I have a client who says that, I wish I could help them find their home. Home could also imply being with a much-missed loved one. I wish I knew which "home" Mom was referring to.

- We have found six of her missing pants. As it is in a memory care unit, things disappear. I had bought a few pairs of pants for her at Lands' End and was upset that so many of them were missing. The staff found them in four different rooms, and all is right with the world again.

- She received some cards for Valentine's Day from two longtime friends, Marilyn and Ardis. Something so simple means so much. We have hung them up in her room so that every day she will remind me she got some cards. Every day continues to be new.

- As a special surprise, I bought her some Girl Scouts cookies from my friend Leslie. Mom was a Girl Scouts leader (Troop 81) when I was a young girl so, besides her love of Thin Mints and lemon cookies, there is some history there. She was excited to get them.

- She voiced missing my dad today. Boy, I second that. I miss having him answer my questions.

- The other comment she has been making is "Well, it's time for bed." This is said at nine in the morning, two in the afternoon, and right before she is going to bed. She has always been an early riser and gave 100 percent the whole day. She loved walking. When I look back in her journals, she really walked even when it rained. I think that is the reason she was in such good shape for almost eighty-eight years old. In the last few months, she has been sleeping more. I catch her in the chair or tucked sweetly in bed, sound asleep. She has found a new love, her bed.

- I am proud that I have not put my mom's roommate's daughter in a headlock. She just can't help making comments about what I buy for Mom. There was another Snickers comment today and I let it go. I was once again glad that she couldn't hear the thoughts in my head. I hope she finds Mom's Girl Scouts cookies.

- Lastly, Mom is worried about her birdhouse outside. It's snowing and she can hardly see it. I tell her it will be fine but I know she doesn't hear me. She's tired and I know her bed is calling. She tells me to go home due to the snow.

The List of Fifty, March 2014

Both of us have had an up-and-down last few weeks. Today I wrote a list of all the things that have been on my mind and some things that I worry about daily. I'm sure the list could be much longer.

1. Does today count? What you do today counts, no matter the memory or lack thereof.

2. When they do not recognize you, know that you are still in their brain history. As hard as it is, you may be lost just for this day.

3. There is a silver lining to the disease; you just need to find it. My time with her is my silver lining.

4. Look at your loved one's hands and know how much they have accomplished in their lives.

5. God is always with Mom. She was a devoted Lutheran and I always catch her singing softly during their services.

6. I hate this disease.

7. When I am sad, I think of my mom in her bikini top, picking raspberries in our garden.

8. Today was not a good day with Mom's roommate's daughter. I might need a glass of wine.

9.   Even if they don't remember your visit, know that you made the effort to go. Mom told someone she hasn't seen me in months.

10. Ask someone how they are doing. Many of us have parents with Parkinson's, memory loss, or cancer, or parents who are just getting older. To inquire means that you care.

11. It's all right to cry. There are moments when I am sad and it will just hit me. Most times it's in the parking lot after my visit.

12. No day will be the same. Today Mom was cranky even though I brought her sister to see her. We ate in a different dining room, which threw her and added to her confusion.

13. I am so proud we have raised more than $20,000 for our Alzheimer's Walk.

14. Find a neurologist who you connect with and trust. I love Mom's doctor.

15. Your loved one is still here.

16. Know that things will disappear in the memory care unit. I have talked about her remote, her toothpaste, her clothes, and today it was her hand soap.

17. Try to pick your battles. My battle right now is with Medical Assistance and understanding all of it. I never will.

18. Medical Assistance denied Mom this week. Go back to #17.

19. I will never understand how the brain works. She can answer a *Wheel of Fortune* puzzle but can't remember her love of cooking or Sophia's name.

20. Always be nice to the caregivers. There may be issues but they have the hardest job. I did the same thing for four years, before becoming a nurse.

21. The Alzheimer's Association is a great place to ask questions. I have used them for many things.

22. We brought our new dog over to see her and she wasn't thrilled. She loves her two stuffed dogs and I accept that.

23. Trust that you are doing the best you know how. I struggle with this on a weekly basis.

24. My mom is still "Super Mom" and I honor her for those days by being good to her right now.

25. You will find yourself bringing her stuffed animals on your travels with her. Someday I will find this funny. Now I just worry about them getting lost.

26. Bring your children to see your loved one. My girls totally understand Mom's memory loss and I hope this understanding will serve them well. They are also very patient with her, even when she doesn't remember their names.

27. Laugh, even though it really isn't funny.

28. Sometimes I hate to go, and I know other people feel the same way.

29. Bingo in a memory care unit is, by far, the best event.

30. She always enjoys getting cards. Please keep sending them.

31. Snickers and coffee have never killed anyone. Can someone tell that to the roommate's daughter?

32. Anger. You are totally allowed to have this feeling.

33. Never state, "Do you remember when or this?" I know how I feel when I don't remember something. Imagine their memory loss and not being able to keep up. And in all fairness, I have forgotten #33 a few times.

34. I have a love/hate relationship with the drug companies. They say it's not a "cure all" medication but they almost make you feel guilty if you don't have your loved one taking them. Mom has been on Namenda and Aricept over the years and I haven't seen one ounce of difference with her memory. But yet I keep her on them and am scared to take her off of them. And boy, do those companies make a lot of money.

35. She can forget who I am. But what bothers me most is the loss of her love for reading, Scrabble, word puzzles, books, and writing letters. I hate that her love of reading is almost gone.

36. If you are worried about your loved one's driving, please have them tested.

37. We misplace the remote five times a week. Where does that thing go?

38. Holidays are hard and Easter is coming. Mom gets overwhelmed with the people and not knowing where she is. This year, sadly, I may just celebrate

with her at Clare Bridge. I hate that because holidays were her favorite time to cook and entertain.

39. She doesn't cook anymore. That almost bothers me as much as her not reading.

40. You feel guilty about everything. It's almost as bad as with my kids. Am I completely screwing up her bills, taxes, paperwork, or life? I don't think that ever goes away.

41. Remember, they had a busy life before their loss happened. I was looking through her 35 mm pictures this week, finishing a project. She looked so beautiful in her bathing suit, holding a stringer of fish. We have over 1,000 pictures of their happy life, before kids. I am having the pictures converted to a CD for her to look at.

42. Sometimes a hug helps. When she is so confused and not having a great day, I hug her and she calms down. We could all benefit from a hug.

43. Have patience. Some days are better than others regarding that.

44. When people come to see her, I try to tell her their names first. That way she is not embarrassed if she doesn't remember their names.

45. Coffee, in large amounts.

46. When you have a large network of friends and family, you have hit the jackpot. I am thankful for the people who help us.

47. I become unglued when I order her briefs from Amazon and see how much they cost. Why didn't I invent adult briefs?

48. Never steal from a vulnerable adult. If you do, I will run you over with my car.

49. Tell her that you love her, even if you know she can't understand or hear you.

50. Pray for a cure for this evil disease.

The Smacker, April 2014

Today I get the best laugh. I arrive at Mom's, loaded with bananas, a large bag of Snickers bars, and some new nylons. It's lunchtime and she's surprised to see me. "Oh, it's you!" She looks nice and cozy, her hair is lovely, and she is banging her cup softly for some coffee. My dad used to do the same thing, which mortified Ross, Mom, and me. I remind her that she can ask and not bang her cup. I feel like I am now the mother.

When I get up to go organize her room, she smacks me in the butt. She has been doing this lately and we both laugh, since it's a pretty hard smack. The nurse on duty catches me in the hallway and lets me know that she has been doing that to other residents too. I'm somewhat surprised at this since she would not hurt a fly. The nurse is not scolding; she is just concerned that another resident may think the gesture is not all right and may hit her back. I know that some of her aides have enjoyed her small tap, but the nurse is correct in thinking this may trigger something bigger.

As I come back to the table, Mom's tablemate is sitting down. I see Mom reaching over to smack her on the arm with a strong wind-up. I catch her and remind her that she needs to be gentle. The other woman is much younger than my mom and said she doesn't mind. But the younger woman's mood also changes on a dime, vacillating between happiness, sadness and anger. Mom continues to pat her tablemate's arm, harder than I would like.

After Mom is done with her meal, I sit down with her and try to explain this smacking business. Again, I feel I'm in the wrong role. I don't really want to have this conversation. It goes something like this:

Me: Mom, you have to be careful when you grab, slap, or smack people. They may not know that you are just being friendly.

Mom: Where is my coffee?

Me: Did you hear me? It's all right to smack me on the butt but try not to do it to someone else.

Mom: Well, it's time for me to get to bed. (It's now 12:30 p.m.)

Me: Mom, don't smack Janet, all right? You know who Janet is; she sits right by you.

Mom: Is that applesauce?

Me: Oh boy, this went well.

Keep in mind, the nurse was just concerned, as am I. In Mom's building, there are many men and some very strong women. When she first arrived, someone pulled her down to the floor. In my experience, I know that this can occur quickly. I am hoping it was an accident.

My visit today is short. I've got so many errands to run.

As I get up to hug her, she pinches my chin. I can tell she notes my surprise. She says, "You said I can't hit you!"

Oh, Mom. How I love you.

The Words

Last week we got the green light from the building to move Mom into a different room. I had put in a request last month because I couldn't take the criticism of the other daughter anymore. Clare Bridge graciously found a room for her on the other side of the building. The room looks exactly the same and she is now near the nursing station and she has a lovely new roommate with a family I have already met. I cannot begin to tell you how relieved I am to move Mom. I can only wish the best for her old roommate's family.

I continue to find it hard with our busy schedules to figure out a time when all three of us can visit. Today it's just the girls and me, each of whom is bringing something for Mom, and I'm excited to show them her new room and have them meet her sweet roommate.

When we arrive, Mom is in the bathroom with an aide and I can tell she's not having a good day. The aide is gentle and sweet with her but I can see a worried expression on her face. She quietly mouths to me, "Your mom wants to die!" Mom is sweaty, nervous, and scratching her back. She is out of sorts.

When I moved Mom on Thursday, everything went very well. As I was leaving that day, the woman from the beauty shop stopped me and asked if everything was all right with Mom. I said she was doing well and told her about the move. She told me that while fixing Mom's hair, she kept saying, "I just want to die." She told me it really bothered her and she even told the nurses she was concerned about her. Mom was normally very funny, a little sarcastic, and never made a fuss getting her hair done.

I had forgotten about the comment until today. She is now out of the bathroom and playing with Matilda, her stuffed dog. She has forgotten the girls' names. I gently remind her and she seems a little better. It's getting to be time for supper and my family heads down the hallway. Mom decides she needs to go back to the bathroom and I take her. While we are in there, she again says, "Why won't God just take me?" and "I just want to die." She is quiet and I can tell the fog of this disease is coming over her. She is confused about why I am here. I slip into nursing mode and ask her questions that she can't answer. Do you hurt? Are you hungry? Did you take a nap today? None of the questions she can answer. As she sits there, she looks at me and pats my face and gives me the biggest sigh.

We leave her room and she is confused about supper. I walk with her and I feel sad. Really sad. We get to her chair after moving people around and she is so quiet. My kids have kissed her goodbye and I can tell the visitor is watching me across the table. She is the sister of a woman who sits with Mom, and I don't want to converse with her. She watches as warm tears are flowing down my face and I'm mortified they have started. I kiss Mom goodbye and walk out to the desk. I catch the evening nurse and ask her to watch over Mom. Again, I cry. I am more of a mess than my mother.

Those words are very powerful. From anyone that you have deeply loved, you really are never prepared for those words. I asked Steve when we got home, "What does she have to live for?" I don't mean to be insensitive, but look at our lives and what her life was. Family, my dad, our activities, church, choir, gardening, and her beloved grandchildren. There was never a time she wasn't doing something.

The previous Thursday, the activity aide had come into her room, inviting her to attend a "Cooking from Scratch" class. I encouraged Mom to go since this is what she did best. Again, she said no. She would rather stay in her room. Life for her has slowed down to a crawl, or even stopped. It's hard for me to accept. In a way, she is even more accepting of it than I am because she has forgotten.

We get home tonight and there is a message to call my aunt, Mom's sister. She is a comfort and we talk about not having Mom come to Easter and that I will most likely just go there instead. We talk about what Mom keeps telling me and how hard it is to hear.

I think that God is not ready for her just yet. I try to find the best in my days with her but today has been a hard day.

The Anger, May 2014

It's about 5 p.m. and I have just gotten home from work. The phone rings and it's one of the nurses from Clare Bridge. "Your mom has not had a good day and she is running a temp. She is also lethargic and her urine is strong. We need to send her to the hospital and I need to know where you want her sent."

I am trying to take in her statement, especially since it's a surprise and I'm still returning work calls from home. I ask the nurse if she really feels we need to send her in and she says yes, she thinks my mom should be evaluated. I agree to send her to the local hospital and I call Steve to let him know I have to leave right away. My mind is going in a million directions since I did not see this coming. It takes me about twenty minutes to get there.

As you can imagine, the hospital visit was not ideal for her. It's a strange place, strange people, she doesn't know why she is there, and they are doing things to her that they should not be doing. They are attempting to put a catheter in her to get a sample of urine and I quickly understand that she thinks they are violating her. I'm trying to explain to her what is going on and she is terrified and crying. Twice she has asked me, "Why are you allowing them to kill me!" This is the reason I do not like to send a confused patient into the ER. They are alone, family can't be with them for whatever reason, and it just doesn't go well. I was glad I could be there and try to help the staff. I hope we never have to do that again. For both of our sakes.

That trip to the emergency room on Thursday made me think of something I have been meaning to write about for so long. It's been in the back of my head, waiting for a time to put it down and for me to articulate it in the best way. It's the way we treat our elderly. Simply put, we need to do better. Not all of us, mind you. Just those who feel it's okay to take advantage of, steal from, or mistreat them.

What happened to Mom in the hospital did not qualify for that kind of mistreatment. I was at the hospital most of the day Thursday and a lunch tray did not arrive for her. I asked the nurse and she said that we needed to order it. My first thought was, how in the world could my mom, being so ill, order her tray or even remember that she needed to order it? I ordered it for her and she only took one bite of her food. I spent the rest of the day trying to get her to eat, with no luck. I left to go home for a while. I had debated not going back since I didn't get home until 2 a.m., but Emme wanted to go back to the hospital and I thought Emme could get her to eat.

We arrived at 7:30 p.m. and Mom was in a fetal position in her bed, a tray sitting on a table by her door. The dinner had not been opened and it was ice cold. I went to sit her up in bed and saw that her IV had infiltrated and her hand was three times the size it should be. As you can imagine, I was less than happy. I found the charge nurse, who said this was not her patient. I told her about what I found and that someone needed to take care of her ASAP. Immediately, we have four nurses in her room and they want to cut off her wedding band, which is sixty-eight years old. I don't want them to do this and I tell them that I will massage her hand to see if some of the fluid will go down. I am furious.

I called the social worker in the morning and asked that Mom be moved back to her memory care unit, hoping she would do better in a place she was more familiar with. I told her I am unhappy with Mom's care. She said she understood and would let someone know. For a week, the "complaint manager" and I played phone tag, but when I finally got to speak to her I told her my concerns. Imagine that you arrive at the hospital to see your mother with her hand totally swollen, which means that no one had checked on her for a while, and that no one fed her. I gave her some examples of how to care for an elderly confused patient, including knowing that they can NOT order food on their own. Her response was to use my mom as a "case study." Do you really need a case study of how to take better care of someone? Can you imagine if I had not gone to see her? I did not tell her I was a registered nurse and the director of our home care agency until the end of the conversation.

I write about this because I have a strong burning anger of how we treat our elderly. I think this was mild compared with what I have seen in the last six months as a nurse, and it sets me on fire. Taking advantage of the elderly must stop. I have been working on a case with a detective to catch a private caregiver who took financial advantage of a woman. I asked her how we can stop this and she said that she sees forty cases a week of elder abuse. That is forty cases a week she actively works on. How can this be? She and I agree that people find an "in" and they take advantage.

I have witnessed theft, getting a vulnerable adult to sign a check, phone call scams, and verbal abuse. I am a mandated reporter, which is someone who looks out for vulnerable people and must make reports to Adult Protection as needed. I make the reports and am told they will not proceed. You almost need to impair or injure someone for it to be looked at. A police officer I spoke to months ago said it's not worth it to prosecute because it's not considered a felony. I don't get it. How do you measure worth?

I have thought about this a lot. You know how we can stop this?

Be nosy and involved. Sure, scams can happen to anyone. But ask and listen when your elderly loved one speaks. I remember after my dad died, a long-term-care insurance company stopped by my mom's house. Her confusion was just starting and she told me some strange man stopped by to visit with her. She said she signed something but she had his number. I called the company and had a direct conversation with the manager about the fact that you can't go door to door and sell that type of insurance. I remember being so angry. They canceled the policy and I wrote a letter to the president of the company.

Red flags: The big thing that's happening with seniors is scams. Guess what! You won a car, but you will need to pay for the taxes on the car, which amounts to $5,000. Guess what! You have won $100,000, but we will need $2,000 as a down payment. And seniors pay it, not knowing any better.

I'm glad for some of my close relationships with my clients because they alert me to things. One client I've had for ten years was scammed on selling her time-share. If your loved one comes to you with these stories, please investigate what they are telling you. I hate hearing these stories because they believe they have won the money. I have a close family friend, my mentor in nursing school, who got bilked out of a dollar amount that would surprise you. He truly believed he would get his money back. The people who call are so sneaky. They say they will arrive with the car or money and it just never arrives and they give you a story that seems plausible. It never is.

I could go on for a long time but I'll stop. Imagine your mother, father, or favorite uncle or aunt. Your older neighbor or your family friend. We must do better to look after them and simply care.

The Mother

One of the hardest jobs is being a mom. But it's something that I'm the most proud of. There is nothing like hearing your child call you Mom for the first time.

I was going through my mom's pictures today and found this sweet one. It was taken two months after I was adopted. It was a happy moment for both my mom and dad, but maybe not so much for my brother. I love the joyful look on her face.

I saw Mom yesterday and we are going through a new stage. She is irritable and crabby with the staff. I can't tell if she doesn't feel good or if she is just mad at everyone. I tell her that I will get her ready for bed and I want to spend a quiet moment with her. When she used to stay with me, it was one of my favorite things to do with the girls, getting Grandma ready for bed.

Her new phrase continues to be "I just want to go to bed." Over and over and over. Trying to distract her, I ask what she wants for Mother's Day. Without hesitation, she states, "I want my mother." I'm surprised by this and I ask her if she remembers what her mother's name is. "Helena Margretha Gertrude Anderson." Wow, she remembered all four names, though I'm not 100 percent sure they are in the right order. I tell her that her mother is not here and that she was gone long before I was born. I can tell this news makes her very sad. "Really?" I say, "Yes, but I've heard that she was a wonderful mother." That seemed to calm her. Can you imagine forgetting that your own mother has died?

As you can imagine, Mom was a good mother. She taught me many things that I'm sure have shaped me as a mother. She showed me how important it was to be kind to someone and to help if you were able. She showed me how to get quiet by picking up a good book. She was always helping someone by baking desserts or homemade bread. I will never be the baker she was. She was the referee, healer, constant taxi driver, peacemaker, lawyer, and chef of our family. She is deeply loved.

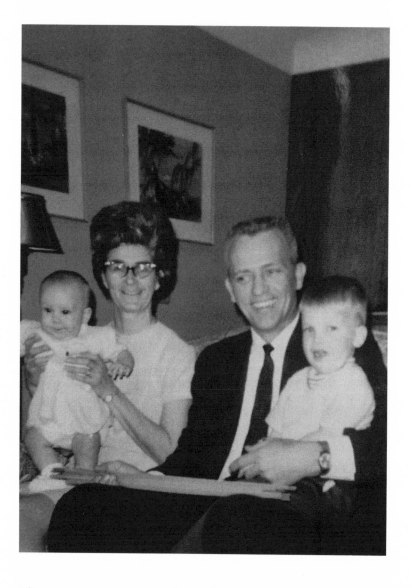

The Rhubarb Queen

When I started my blog, many names for it came to mind. The Rhubarb Queen was at the top of the list. I think both The Lemon Bar Queen and The Rhubarb Queen are accurate in describing my mom. She is one of the best bakers I know.

Rhubarb has been a part of our household for as long as I can remember. When I was growing up on our farm, we had huge rhubarb plants. Every spring my mom taught me how to cut the stalks, reminding me not to take the small ones and to leave the giant woody ones. She also used the leaves as compost in our garden. I remember my dad putting coffee grounds on the base of the plants and they grew to be lush and enormous. It seems like yesterday that Mom would put on her old yellow shorts (that she sewed herself), her top with the sleeves cut off, and a scarf pulling her hair back, her legs always with a farmer's tan.

Just the smell of rhubarb brings me back. Mom loved to cut it up for jam, muffins, torte, bread, sauce, and our favorite, pie. It was always a treat to have vanilla ice cream with warm rhubarb sauce steaming over the top. My love affair with this strange plant started young.

When my parents moved from the farm and bought a house in town, along came the rhubarb. They transplanted it on the side of the house. The canning and baking continued.

Fast-forward twenty-five years.

I've shared that my mom isn't eating that much since returning from the hospital. Just eating enough to keep a bird alive. I have tried to get her to eat more. Snickers bars, cheeseburgers with fried onions, cashews, Snickers Blizzards, cookies. She only takes a few bites and even refuses her beloved coffee. I'm frustrated. So is she. She doesn't understand why it's so important that she eat. Her new favorite phrase is repeated over and over: "I want to die!"

I decided to buy some rhubarb last week. I skimmed her well-worn church cookbook, *The Fron Cookbook*. I turn to page 198, which is dog-eared, to find Rhubarb Dessert by Mrs. Russell Lundell. So I decide to make her dessert. The whole house fills with the lush smell of rhubarb and I am so excited to bring her a

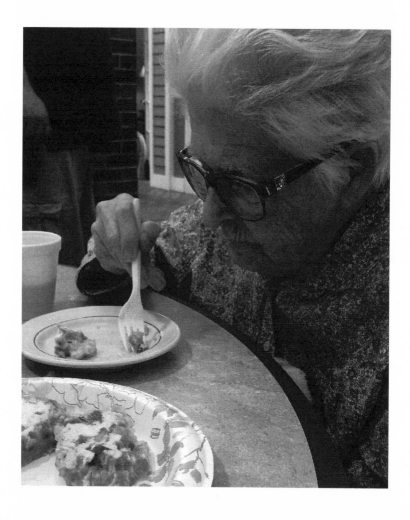

piece. On a side note, my ten-year-old is limited in how much she eats because last year she ate so much dessert that she vomited in the middle of the night. That is a mess you can never unsee and I had to clean it up by myself since Steve was dry-heaving at the thought of helping.

When I bring over her dessert, she is sitting in their parlor area and she smiles and waves at me. I'm hoping that this very special gift will get her to eat. I told her I would get her some coffee and we could share a piece. I see a small glimmer in her eye and she asks for a fork. This is a good sign. She grabs the fork and takes a small bite and then a sip of coffee. She looks up at me and I can tell she likes it. Bite after bite she finishes the whole piece. She even finishes her coffee. I am thrilled and feeling victorious. I even bribed her with another piece of dessert to get her hair done. (For some reason, she has been annoyed with getting her hair done, a new behavior that I am unsure of.) For the past week, I have been researching rhubarb recipes. My friend Dawn made the best scones, called Naughty Rhubarb Scones, so Sophia and I made them over the weekend. I brought them to Mom's yesterday and she thought they were a bit strange, but she ate the whole thing. Success yet again.

Today I was up at five a.m., thanks to our dog, Barley. Not being able to get back to sleep, I made Mom's dessert and brought some to school for the staff. I am reminded that I most likely did the same thing as Mom did, all those long years ago. She would get up early to bake. I'm sure it was her time while we were sleeping. She was alone and enjoying what she loved to do the most, bake. My next project will be rhubarb crisp with some vanilla ice cream. I'm hoping she will respond as she did with my last experiment.

Rhubarb. Who knew that this magical plant would help my mom at this stage in her life? I will never be the cook my mother was. It was her joy and I can think of a hundred things I would rather do than bake. But for her, I can attempt this one time a week, and Sophia has enjoyed helping, just like I did as a child.

The Other Slapper, June 2014

The last few weeks have been some long ones for Mom and me. This disease is one that changes daily, so we have good days and difficult days.

I was at work last Friday assessing a woman with dementia. She had been leaving her stove on and getting up in the middle of the night looking for her dead husband. Sometimes the people I assess mimic my own situation and the things Mom does.

I think about this disease every day. If I'm not at work, I'm signing papers, picking up medications, fighting with Medicare, going through bills, or taking Mom to an appointment. She needed a follow-up appointment today because the hospital doctor would not sign off on her physical therapy, so the girls and I picked her up and took her to see Dr. Graham. She is a wonderful doctor who works with Dr. Woodland and who understands this terrible disease. She would also be the doctor that let Mom hold Blue Dog during an X-ray. That is something you can't teach in medical school.

When I completed assessing this woman, I went back to my car and saw that I had two missed calls from Mom's memory care unit. The messages sounded urgent. My heart started to beat faster and I knew I would most likely not receive the best news. I called the nurse right away. Mom was slapped across the face by another resident. I can feel the air rush out of me and my heart sink.

Apparently, the woman grabbed my mom's lunch tray, which my mom was not very happy about, so she told her to give it back and the woman, with an open hand, slapped her on the cheek and pushed her chair. The incident was witnessed and the woman removed.

I thought about this incident as a daughter first and then as a logical nurse. It brings me back to the days when I worked in the memory care unit in the nursing home. We were hit almost every day and we prevented people from getting hit. It was a constant battle sometimes. When people can't communicate, they act out by hitting, which is what I think this woman did.

This woman, just like Mom, is a mother, sister, friend, cousin, and human being. I imagine her family is also dreading a call. It may be even worse on their end, knowing that their loved one hurt someone else. It could also be my own mother hitting someone and not just smacking people on the butt.

I almost feel like that mother on the playground who watches another child hit her own in some battle. Your inner "Momma Bear" comes out, or in this situation, daughter. Today I saw the woman and I could tell she was having a hard day again. I waved to her and have come to peace with her. She can't help it, just like my mom can't help saying over and over that she wants to go to bed and to die. I will add this woman to my thoughts and prayers and we will move on. I will keep an eye on her, though.

The Roommate, July 2014

Just for today, I'm not writing about Mom. I'm writing about her roommate. I have just come back from a well-needed break with my family and I have not talked to my mom in over a week. I know she is well cared for and I have only worried about her a little, though I have missed our banter. My brother was in charge while we were gone.

Today after work, I headed to Mom's to bring her a treat. The good thing about memory loss is that I don't think she even remembered I was gone. She gave me a big smile. I told her we went to the lake and I showed her the video of Sophia getting up on water skis. She said that she needed to get to bed, and so we went.

I opened her bedroom door and waved to her roommate. I did not get a response. I brought Mom to her chair and I went over to say hello to her. I could tell right away she had had a stroke and I wiped the drool from her face. Half of her face gave me a smile. There was a lone chair sitting by her bed that someone had most likely used today.

I don't know much about Mom's new roommate but I know that she is beautiful, sweet, well dressed, and always worried about Mom, especially when she came back from the hospital.

I love to see her pictures on the wall of a much different-looking woman: cheeks heavier, hair high and very blonde, standing with her handsome husband. I know that her sister has faithfully taken her out for lunch every Thursday. Her life, like Mom's, is vastly different than it used to be.

My girls quickly formed a pact that they would pretend to be her grandchildren. They would come into her room and shout hello to her. Sophia would sit in her chair while she was in bed and they would discuss Mom. I loved the little relationship they formed with her. I think children are always a highlight for the elderly, remembering days that have long passed and how much noise they make, especially my girls.

I don't think Mom could have found a better roommate. I also have enjoyed my time with her. I always gave her a mini Snickers out of Mom's supply. Twice, I've seen her fall while I was in the room. She was a sneaky one, transferring herself into bed when she should have waited. One time, she would have broken her wrist, but I saw her out of the corner of my eye and picked her up right away. It's just an instinct to help, even though I shouldn't be doing that at Mom's place. I scolded her kindly and told her she has to wait. No more falls.

Now her beautiful face is pale and drooping. And she is coughing, and no one is around. It reminds me of my nursing home days and wanting to be everywhere but not being able to. I get her nurse and they help her get comfortable, my mom not even realizing what's going on. For a brief moment, I get to hold her hand. It's always hard for me when someone's family is not there and I'm the only person with them. Knowing that her time is limited, I hope she can get comfortable quickly.

Life changes so quickly. Eight days ago my girls saw their grandma before vacation and got to talk to their grandma's roommate, a kind and gentle woman who I hope finds peace and her handsome husband soon.

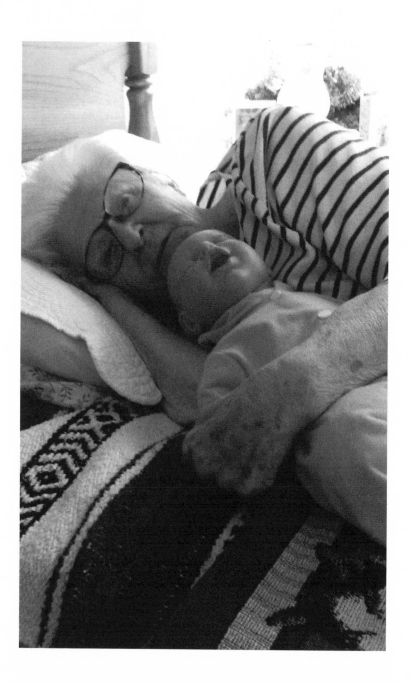

The Baby, July 2014

If you look closely at this photo, you can see my mom smiling. It's a rare smile and it's a good sign. She is happy.

When Sophia and I went to see her today, we found her with a baby doll. Last Tuesday at the barbecue they hosted at her memory care unit, she also had a baby doll. It was sitting on her walker, naked and a little beat up. She introduced me to her baby and I put it on a chair, hoping she would forget about it. The week before, I had called her at night and when she finally answered the phone she said she was in bed and snuggling with her baby. I thought she meant her stuffed dog, Matilda. What she was really talking about was this new addition. The Baby.

Honestly, I am not thrilled with this new addition. I have gotten used to her talking to her animals and mainly her dog. We take the animals with us when we go on our trips and appointments, and I have gotten used to their presence. They do bring her comfort and joy. Now she has Matilda the crazy-haired dog, a blue stuffed dog with no name, and a hockey bear that she also cuddles with. And now a baby.

It's difficult for me to see my mom holding this baby. I know logically that it brings her some joy. Working in the nursing home and in home care, I see many elderly with their most-loved items. When I worked in the memory care unit, it varied from a suitcase, to a baby doll, a blanket, and a purse. I know the items bring something familiar to them, especially when most everything else is taken away.

But as I look at this doll, it represents where Mom is in her loss. She is comforted by a heavy, plastic, very real-looking doll. I asked her today, "Do you know that the doll is fake?" Her answer was a simple "Yes." She then began to talk to it and offer it a bite of banana that we brought for her. I think Sophia, my soon-to-be eleven-year-old, handled it better than I did. She asked Mom questions and we found that she named the baby Jodi. I am secretly thrilled she named it after me.

My mother, now with her baby, is content and smiled today. I understand her memory loss, but it's hard for me to realize she is finding comfort in this. It's hard for me to put this into words. But when I see her talk to the baby, I feel her loss. She is talking to a lifelike baby that weighs ten pounds. I need to accept that she loves this fake baby.

Before we leave, I go into the nursery area that they have for the residents and I trade out her baby for a lighter-weight doll. Sophia and I put a different outfit on her, and Mom doesn't even realize it's a different baby. She snuggles right in with it and gives it a kiss and then tells Sophia, "I think I'm too rough with it!"

We leave after a long visit and she tells me she loves us both and she waves the baby's hand at us. This baby thing is going to take me a while to get used to.

On the car ride home, I think that she is just holding me when she holds that baby. She may be going back forty-plus years and holding what she thinks is me, and I must understand that. If the baby is a reflection of me, I'm all right with that. I guess.

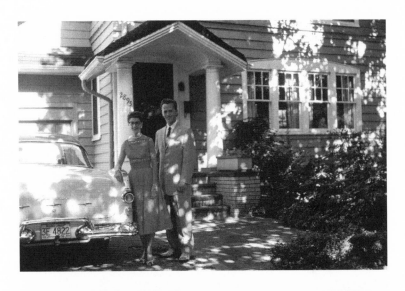

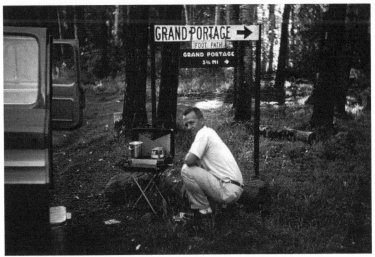

The Father, August 2014

Tomorrow marks seven years that my father has been gone. It's a day I normally bring up with Mom so that she still remembers his name and image. I can hardly believe he has been gone that long.

There is not one day that goes by that I don't think of him. In Mom's room, I keep a great picture of him right by her bed. I have also hung their wedding picture above her bed. They were married on August 16 and if he were still alive it would have been their 67th anniversary.

I caught her playing with her ring the other day and she asked me about mine. Our rings are both platinum and she likes to twist mine on my finger, questioning who gave it to me. I asked her last week, "Who gave you your ring?" She looked at it and twisted it around on her finger. "Oh, I guess Russell did." I am grateful she remembers. They had many ups and downs in their life, but they managed to stay together, and I miss him a lot.

I regret that he never got to meet Emme. I miss that he hasn't been able to see Sophia play baseball. If he were here, he would be yelling at the ballpark, giving pointers and we would bring him to the ice rink to watch the girls play hockey. I miss his wisdom and advice, whether I wanted to hear it or not. He was a complex man, but his wisdom was normally right on.

He loved my mother very much, and the day before he died is etched in my mind. I remember that conversation from his bed in his den as he detailed his concerns about Mom and her memory loss. After seven years of watching her finances, I know that her money comes to an end next month and I will apply for medical assistance. For the second time, since I was denied in December because she had too much money to qualify.

I feel my dad around me sometimes and I continue to ask him questions, even though I don't get a response. I feel like sometimes I'm making a mistake, and I long for him to tell me to try a different way. I was thinking of him Friday when I didn't make the best nursing judgment of being alone with a client in a hotel room, setting up the client's medications. He had been kicked out of a nursing home and we were hired to set up medications until he could find placement. I felt uncomfortable. We got on the subject of my dad because they were both engineers, and I felt my Dad watching over me to make sure I was safe. If he were alive, I know that he would have called me a knucklehead, just like he used to, and would've reminded me to use my head.

I wish I could just hear him call my name. I so miss hearing that. I hope he's proud of the way I've taken care of Mom. Grief never goes away. It's always there—sometimes a small black cloud hanging over your head deciding if it should rain on you or not. I'm sometimes glad that Mom may forget the pain of losing him. A rare good thing about her memory loss.

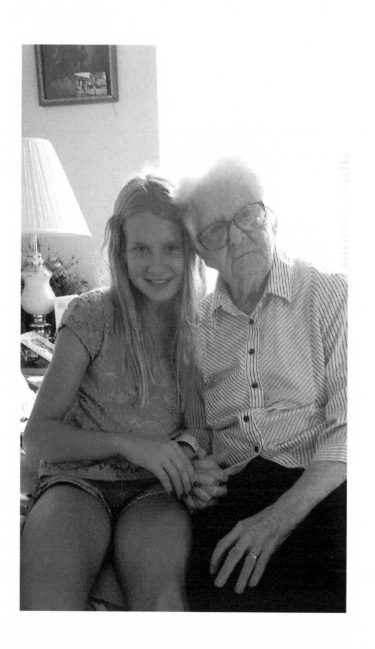

The Cry, August 2014

This picture was taken last week, upon our return from vacation. I love that they are holding hands and that for that day Mom remembered Sophia's name. They chatted like they normally do and she got to slap Sophia's bare legs, which has been her recent way of communication. We also brought her a big cupcake from Gigi's and I think she was in heaven.

Fast-forward to last night and her small stroke. I've noticed that things happen when you are the busiest. Yesterday was the first day of school and I was up early. Work was busy and I got to try a new fitness class after work. When I finally noted missed calls on my phone from Steve, I learned that Mom had a stroke.

Stroke.

I found her sitting in a chair, glasses crooked and her beautiful face drooping on the left side. Her first words? "Where have you been?" I laughed. Her speech is garbled but I can understand her. The nurse gives me a quick update but I can clearly tell she's had a stroke. Just when I finally got her to eat and she's back on track from her hospital stay, we have a setback.

I ask her if she can walk with me and I can feel myself assessing her. She is weaker on her left side but able to walk. As we walk through her doorway, she notices the ceramic church she painted that looks like her hometown Lutheran church, and I ask the staff if I can get her ready for bed. She slaps my bare thighs and I know she is feeling better after the slow walk.

She is a little confused and she asks, "What's wrong with me?" I tell her she has had a small stroke and that her speech is a little goofy right now. She asks me to scratch her back and I can tell she is tired. We finish her nightly routine in the bathroom and I get her into bed. I notice her eyes are not as wide open anymore and her speech is worse as she gets into bed with her baby. She pats my face and softly states, "Thank you for helping me." I can understand that jumbled speech. Even in her confusion, she is thankful. I haven't cried since I arrived but I can feel the tears start. She watches me and also starts to tear up. She murmurs, "I want to die," over and over and over and over and over.

I haven't seen my mom cry since my dad died, seven years ago. Part of this disease is that it robs people of emotion. She rarely smiles, never cries, and says things that are not appropriate. The filter is gone and so is the ability to show that emotion that I sometimes long for.

I hate that this is happening to her. I feel like we are on a roller coaster with this disease. One thing after another. Highs and lows. Happy and sad. It's exhausting, but I feel I can't complain because it could be worse. Much worse.

I put the picture of my dad right by her bed and tell her he will watch out for her tonight. She stares at it and I wonder if she can see it due to the stroke. The last thing she asks is, "Am I alive?" I tell her yes. "You are not in heaven yet." I'm teasing her, but she doesn't respond. She's already asleep, that quickly.

Today I'm writing this with her. Her speech is still the same. We went for a short walk. I have a call in for her doctor and I'm watching her eat a mini doughnut I brought her. We have another day together.

I tell her that I let my friends and our family know that she's not feeling the best and that they were thinking of her and praying. That seemed to bring her comfort. The journey continues.

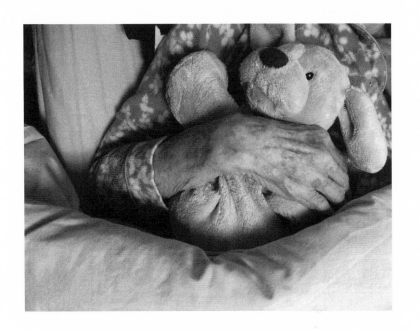

The Forty-Fourth Year,
September 2014

The stroke continues to affect her left side and her speech. Her speech is slowly coming back, but she's tired and weaker. I made the difficult decision to start hospice care last Thursday. She is still loving and funny, just weaker. She still slaps my butt every time she catches me or the girls. I catch a half smile from her when she does.

This has been strange for me, being on the other end of hospice care. My background has been cardiac care and more recently home care and hospice. It was strange to answer questions and not be the one asking them. In the past few days I have signed more papers than I can count. I was also on the phone with the economic assistance program and Department of Aging for three hours last week. We ordered a new wheelchair, discontinued some medications, spoke to the bath aide, encouraged a pastor visit and music therapy, and requested a massage, and I finally spoke to the social worker.

All through this, my friends and family have helped me, mainly my husband, Steve. He has been my rock through all of this. My girls have taken her for walks, gotten her ready for bed, scratched her back, and given her Ensure. I'm so proud of them. Here's hoping one of them will decide on a career in medicine. They can take care of Steve and me when we get old.

Today I am meeting with a social worker and she asks me to describe Mom. I sit and look at this simple piece of paper and think of how I can articulate Mom's life.

I want this social worker to know that she loves toast and

cheese and that she made doughnuts from scratch. I want her to know that I taught her how to drive a stick shift in her mid-sixties and how it took forever for her to learn on that old tan Ford Escort. One of my very favorite memories of our time together as mother and daughter.

I want her to know that she tried for twenty years to have children. I'm sure watching her brothers, her sister, and her friends have babies and being unable to conceive was hard on her. I want her to know that she finally got a boy and girl and how much she adored us. You don't have to carry a baby for nine months to be a mother. She loved starting the day with coffee and a long walk. She did leg kicks and stretches in the morning to stay fit. Mom loved playing the slot machines in Yuma, but only playing the nickels. Mom helped with Girl Scouts, Sunday School, and Bible Choir and loved spending time with Sophia and Emme. She always said she waited a lifetime for those two, and we have fifty quilts to prove it.

The social worker needs to know that even when Mom was starting to get more forgetful, she would still remember to send me stamps in the mail and buy Steve white tube socks. I tell the social worker how much she loves Steve and all of her nieces and nephews. Before her memory loss, always sending a card with a little money in it to her family.

My parents were married for sixty years, and during that time she traveled, hunted for mushrooms, canned everything and anything, searched for agates, entertained friends, helped with reports, and looked for my shoes at night so she knew that I finally was home safe and sound.

I want to share with her that Mom read at night, hummed while she baked, was afraid of snakes, and once killed a bat with a tennis racket. She loved being tan, was a devout Lutheran, and never pierced her ears.

Lastly, I want her to know what a good mother she is. Always helping, always busy, always caring, and always loving. It's hard to sum up your mother on one sheet of paper. She could also make anything out of rhubarb, and her lemon bars are amazing.

She and I have been together forty-four years. I am so lucky.

The Day Off, October 2014

Today has not been a good day for Mom. We sat on her bed this afternoon and talked about what was bothering her. She's a little winded and I'm not quite sure she knows it's me. Here's what she's trying to tell me:

> "I feel 'cheesy' inside."
> "I wish I could die." (100+ times)
> "I've got to get to work ... I need to get to work ...
>   It's my work day."
> "I've got to get to bed."
> "Are you tired of me?"

She is out of sorts about "work," which is new. I try to calm her down and tell her it's her day off and that they don't need her. I also let her know it's Saturday. You know what helped? Sophia.

This picture says a lot. They are holding hands while Mom looks so sad. It speaks volumes about this disease. I really can't make it all go away. But my soon-to-be eleven-year-old can, for just a while. They talk a little and she is calmer. I wonder if she thinks Sophia is me at a younger age. She also has her doll and her blue dog. We lost it for a few days but when we arrived today, there Blue was sitting, waiting for us on the piano. Sophia said it was like magic, finding it right there.

There are many reasons to hate this disease. Watching Mom so worried about getting to work was very difficult for me. Something must have triggered in her brain that made her think she had to go to work. She's always been a hard worker.

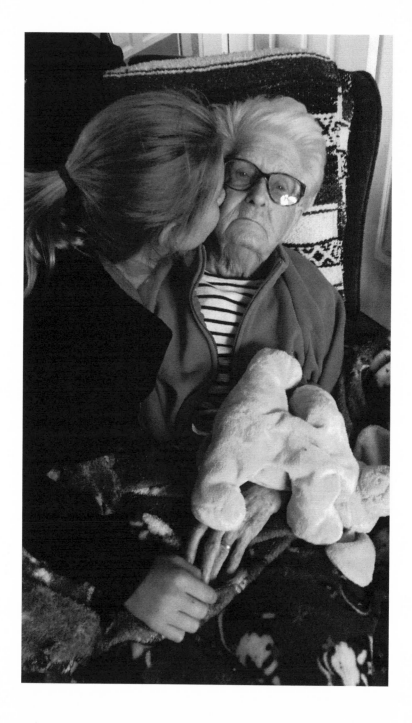

The Feeder Table

After Mom's stroke, the staff asked if they could move her to a feeder table and I agreed. She wasn't able to get her food on the fork and it was becoming a struggle for her and for us to watch. I feel the same way about her wheelchair as I do the feeder table. Just watching her decline is an ache that is constant.

So tonight I sit on these hard, unforgiving chairs, surrounded by staff and other people, feeding my mother. For supper tonight, it is sloppy joes, green beans, hash browns, and a fresh-baked cookie. For a treat I have brought her pumpkin bread and a cookie. I know if she refuses her regular food, I can always get her to eat a treat with coffee.

I know that she loves green beans; she grew a huge garden filled with them. The meal smells so good, but she is refusing most of it. I try to get her to eat and she shakes her head no. I nod my head yes. She shakes her head no. And so on and so on. I get her to eat the pumpkin bread and she nearly finishes it.

As I sit here, I can hardly believe I'm feeding my mother. Her mission in life was to feed people. For twenty years she worked for Lutheran Brotherhood, cooking meals for seniors. She would wake up at six in the morning and walk two blocks in all sorts of weather to open the center and make the noon lunch. She loved that job and most likely made thousands of meals in those twenty years. In a small town, people stopped by our house often and she was always ready with a meal in the refrigerator or freezer. She enjoyed making our family wonderful meals. She continued to make meals for funerals, weddings, and people who were ill or needed their spirits lifted. Mom loved being a feeder. It gave her much pleasure. I know that in this world there are feeders. My friends Leanne and Nichol are feeders and so is my mom's sister, Gloria. I'm lucky to get the benefits of them feeding me. They are so much like my mom.

Now I'm the one feeding her one bite at a time. She gives me a look. I know the look. She would rather not have me doing this. I understand and I put the fork down. I let her know that I would bring a burger with fried onions next time. She gives me a slow, sweet smile. I knew that would make her happy. So too would a Dairy Queen Snickers Blizzard.

I get her ready for bed. I haven't seen her in over a week because I've been so busy. Work, the school book fair, Sophia's birthday, and many other projects. I know she doesn't realize I've been away that long, but I've missed her. She looks tired and weak to me. The hospice nurse says she had an okay visit with her.

After I tuck her in, I continue the habit of turning my dad's picture toward her, right by her bed. Tonight she says, "Do you know if he's in the house?" I pause for a second, the comment somewhat surprising me. I tell her, "I think he's always in the house." She gives me a second smile, closes her eyes, and goes to sleep.

The Garage Sale Farmer

Over the last few days, I've had a garage sale to get rid of some items, including my mom's many clothes. Overall the sale went well. Boy, did I meet some people with personalities. One of those people was a man named Stan.

Stan came to the sale looking for men's shirts and the only thing I had was Steve's long black cashmere coat. I had priced it at $5 and we went around and around about it. He wanted to buy it for $2.50. I stuck to my guns and asked $5 for it. He enjoyed that I wouldn't sell it to him.

Stan told me that he was from Clara City and he had walked to my house from his daughter's home. He had retired seven years ago and loved being able to come to town to see his grandkids. He loves to go for walks when he is here and he asked about Steve's work truck. He told me he farmed most of his life but dabbled in construction. He was surprised to hear that I grew up on a farm and we talked about farm life. He asked about my parents and I told him a little about Mom, including how we moved her closer to me. I told him how much I missed my own parents coming to see me, as he is doing with his family. He said his own memory isn't what it used to be. He hoped he didn't get "the disease."

We talked about small towns, his stint in the war, playing horseshoes in Clara City, and how it's a competitive sport where he lives. He broke down all the scoring in great detail, with great pride. I told him my dad taught me how to play many years ago and that we had a horseshoe pit on our farm. He talked about where his grandkids went to school and how proud he was of his daughters and what good mothers they were. He told me about how sad the six-year-old was to leave his mother to go to school, but now he doesn't cry anymore. He said his daughter is also an RN and works for Methodist Hospital. He also bragged about Lake Minnewaska and said what a good lake we had.

Just looking at him, I was reminded so much of my dad. Stan looked about the same age my dad was when he died. Farmer cap, three layers on due to the weather, old weathered jeans, and pointy-toed boots. It was such a breath of fresh air from the people I had met who wanted to pay fifty cents for everything. I must have spent forty-five minutes with him. He finally said he needed to go, as his family was most likely worried about him.

I closed up the garage sale, and sitting there was the coat. No one had bought it. I knew roughly where Stan's family lived and I drove up the road. Some kids were playing in the street and I asked them if they knew where this certain family lived. They pointed to a green house. I knocked on the door and Stan's son-in-law answered holding a baby. He called out for Stan.

He must have known about our conversation because the son-in-law had a big smile on his face. Stan came to the door and I gave him the coat. He asked if I wanted $2.50 for it and I said it was free. He was happy and said, "Thanks, Starbuck girl."

My heart was so full after I left. I think there are people meant to come into your life, maybe just for a moment. I'm not sure what the moment was supposed to mean, but I hope I see him again. It was just like seeing my dad again.

The Word Find, November 2014

Today was the day I was going to take Mom out for a car ride, but it's cold and damp out and I know she won't enjoy it. So I have switched gears and decided to spend the day with her and talk with her hospice nurse, who comes every Thursday.

I went to Costco yesterday and bought a beautiful fall bouquet of flowers and a bag of Halloween candy for her and the staff. She hasn't been following our book reading as of late, so I brought her *Midwest* magazine so she can page through the cookies section.

When I arrive, I find her at the church service, sitting by herself. She gives me a small smile. I can tell she isn't sure who I am, which is happening more and more. She wants to know if the flowers are for her and if her sister sent them. I told her that I bought them for her and she is confused, thinking I am delivering them. I remind her, "It's Jodi, Mom." We sit face-to-face, off to the side, and I can tell I'm coming back to her. I love that moment when she realizes it's me.

I have brought her candy and coffee and we wait for her hospice nurse. There is a lot of activity going on around us. She starts eating a Snickers bar and then grabs a cookie too. I sit by Jean, a woman I used to take care of and who has now moved to memory care. We share cookies and coffee together. It's almost like being at Mom's Circle at her church. We talk a little about Fron Church and how she misses it and the people.

The hospice nurse arrives and we talk about Mom quietly, off to the side. She seems to be shrinking every day, just getting ever so smaller, and her voice is quieter. I think she knows we are talking about her. She asks if she can have the cheese and crackers in front of her. She has started to eat more and I'm surprised but happy to see her enjoying food. I voice my concerns to the nurse. Weight loss, the constant wheelchair, and how she leans to the left all the time. She has also noted how quiet Mom's voice seems. Mom's nurse, Cathy, is a gift. She understands the progression of this disease and answers my questions. She is gentle and kind. I confess to her that I wish my brother would come and see Mom. Mom smiles at her, too, which is wonderful.

Mom is ready for bed at 11 a.m. and I take her to her room and transfer her gently into her chair. She has been having trouble with words today and I catch her staring at me. I am rambling on like I do with her. I am talking about Sophia's hockey and how she made math masters. I am telling her how proud I am of Emme and her reading skills, and we talk about how tomorrow is Halloween. I'm going on and on and she stops me.

"I like you."

I stop talking and look at her. "I like you too, Mom." I know that she was trying to find the word love, but "like" comes out instead. I can tell that she isn't sure who I am again and she looks at the flowers that I put by the bed. I wonder if she still thinks I'm the flower delivery person. I stop telling her about our family "stuff" and we end up lying in her bed, watching Channel 2 before she goes to lunch.

It's hard when Mom forgets me. I know it's normal in the progression of this disease, but try to tell that to my heart. I try to remember how lucky I have it with Mom. She doesn't hit anyone or scream at the staff. She's calm and polite. One of the aides told me last week that Mom is one of her favorites. Teasing, I told her she says that to all the families. She said no and told me why. She said, "No matter what we're doing together, your mom always says thank you." I can imagine they don't hear that often. I love that she shared that with me.

Day 49 of Hospice
Jodi/Flower Delivery Girl

I'm sitting in my car in front of Mom's memory care unit. She is again confused about who I am today, so I have left and am watching people come and go while I'm sobbing in my car. I hate this fucking disease. I know my mom would be appalled that I have used this term. I'm sorry. But it describes this disease that I hate so much. That is all for today.

...but they'll never change
how close we feel.

Thinking of You
at Thanksgiving

Jeanne

The Blessing

Today I got to spend a few hours with Mom at lunchtime. I got a call late last night that she was sick at dinner time and I wanted to see how she was doing today. I also brought her cards to sign for her friends in Starbuck. I have been behind on sending them. Her friends have been so good about sending her cards and little notes. We read them and put them up on her wall.

Today I'm impressed that she wants to sign her name. We practiced a little after lunch so she would get it right. She hasn't had to write her name in a while. Her first attempt was impressive. She just kept forgetting to put the e on the end of her name. In the last attempt she started to write Marie, which is her middle name. She was concerned that her signature looks awful. I explained to her that her friends will not care; they just like hearing from her. She used to take great pride in her handwriting.

We talked about Thanksgiving coming up and I told her I would come and we could eat together. I will most likely bring her a plate from our house. I'm not sure if I could get her in our car or if she would tolerate the ride. I'm reminded of all those wonderful years she cooked a turkey dinner for our family and how those years are now gone from her memory.

Back in her room, she wants to crawl into her bed. I sit in her chair and we watch each other. I think that has been her biggest pastime lately. She just sits and watches me. She has her blue dog, and the aide, Alice, tells me that she has had a good day. Mickey, the activity aide, states that she pinched her butt today. All is good.

As I sit in her brown chair, I think of all the people who have helped me in the last few weeks. I think it's important to acknowledge the people who are such a blessing in your life and how thankful you are for their help.

My mom's hairdresser, who is her "hair advocate," had a fit when she found out hospice washed her hair after she just did it. Without charging Mom, she fixes it when they don't do her hair the way she thinks it should be done. Mom always liked having her hair done.

Mom's new social worker, Sheila, answers complicated questions with ease. On occasion she needs to explain things to me over and over. Medicare, medical assistance, and hospice together is a complicated mess. She is calm and determined, which I love. One day, she and I calculated how many pads my mom would go through, because medical assistance will pay for it. I still think it's funny we are estimating that.

Steve is a volunteer at Clare Bridge every other Wednesday. Staff told me that he adores my mom and looks after her because she reminds him of his own mom. Since my brother has not seen her in a while, I love that she has a male figure she can talk to. I have met him there once, but I don't go on Wednesday nights because it's our church night. I love the fact that he looks after her.

All of my friends ask about her when they see me. I have always felt that to inquire means that you care. All of our parents are getting older and we can all learn from one another's experiences. It's so hard to watch our parents get older.

My neighbor Mary took the girls to Grandfriends Day yesterday. My mom would have loved to go to any school event. I know that she would not want to miss anything if she could help it. The girls' other grandma could not attend so they wanted to ask Mary and she said YES! I know they were proud to have Mary go. Thank you, Mary!

I'm thankful that I get to share my experiences. This week, I was interviewed by a college student regarding hospice care. It's such an important field of nursing and I know that Jessica will get an A on her paper! Good luck, Jessica!

I have said this before but it bears repeating. My mom's hospice nurse is an angel. I am lucky to connect with someone who also provides such loving care to my mother. I love that she always hugs Mom and my mom responds to her.

I'm also thankful that I never started smoking. If I had, I would be up to two packs a day.

I am even thankful for my mom's ex-roommate's daughter. I saw her today at lunchtime. She ignores me and I am all right with that. I'm reminded that it's perfectly all right not to follow rules so closely and that Mom's end-of-life care should be celebrated. Eat candy, have nuts and popcorn, and drink coffee until you can't take another breath. Isn't this disease awful enough to limit what they can enjoy? She still makes me want to have a glass of wine after I see her, though.

I am blessed to have a wonderful husband and two girls who love their mother-in-law and grandma, no matter if she forgets their names. I love the smile that they can get out of her.

Thank you to Sophia's choir director, Barb. She has been organizing Sophia's All District Choir to come sing for Mom and the residents. Sophia sang at Orchestra Hall last week and we were talking about how Mom would have loved to see Sophia sing. We talked about bringing the singers to Mom. And, like magic, we have December 4 on the calendar for a private concert. Isn't that just amazing? I know she will love hearing them sing. Thank you to all who helped plan this.

Lastly, I received a beautiful letter from my dad's side of the family. It was from a cousin of Dad's who lives in Florida and reads my blog. She wrote at the end, "I pray the Lord is with you and your family in the days ahead." Thank you, Phyllis. I hope so too.

The Holiday, December 2014

The great part of my job is the people I get to meet every day. I've had some of my clients for just a few short days; others I've had for years. I get to watch their ups and downs, happy and sad days, joys and grief.

Today was a grief day. My first visit was with a man who just lost his wife four days ago. He is sweet and loving. He lost her suddenly, and his tears spill over as he talks with me this morning. They were married over seventy years and he was her primary caregiver. Suzie, one of our nurses, told me they were screaming "I love you!" when they finally were reunited last Wednesday (they were both hard of hearing). Today he talked about her and the sadness he felt. It's a long time to be with someone, and he told me he isn't interested in the upcoming Christmas holiday. I completely understood.

My next visit was with a woman I am attached to. She is smarter than anyone I know, an avid reader of all things, super intelligent, and respected by many. She says she is a nonpracticing Jew and has taught me about the war in Israel and has broken down for me what each side believes in, all while being nonjudgmental. We discuss audiobooks she is listening to, because her eyesight is poor and fading. I always feel that her reading vastly differs from my fluff reading, but she never judges. I told her all about *The Orphan Train* when I was reading it. She ordered it on audiobook. She taught in Israel and at New York University, and has many students still come to visit her. She keeps me on my visits way too long, but I love to listen to her.

Today, she is very weak and she had a tough weekend. She is waiting for her father to come get her and she tells me right away that there is an intruder in her house with a gun. I tell her I would not be here if there was someone bad in her home. But she doesn't believe me. Her daughter arrives and we both calmly tell her that she is okay and safe. Even with her garbled speech she tells us, "I'm grateful for you both." She also tells us, "I am a slave and need to be set free." That makes the daughter cry. I'm not sure if she will make it to their own family-oriented holiday gathering. It's always hard to say goodbye, but she is in good hands with her family and our staff.

My last visit of the day was with a woman whose apartment is 104 degrees. Okay, maybe 100 degrees. I tell her it's too hot in her apartment but she has been having some side effects of her cancer, making her cold. She has told me for the tenth time that God is not coming for her and that she is ready to go. Like now. She couldn't care less about this upcoming Christmas holiday and wants us to stop fussing over her. She is tiny, forgetful, and a powerhouse of the family. I tell her that I understand, while her daughter just nods her head.

I was talking with my friend Leanne and we both agreed the holidays are hard for people. I could feel everyone's grief today. I think of my own grief of not taking Mom out for Thanksgiving and her own statements of wanting to die. I miss her pumpkin pies, her homemade buns, and listening to her open the oven door and whisk the gravy. Her memories are gone of our family-filled holidays.

All three of today's patients stay with me today and I understand their feelings 100 percent. I'm wishing them peace tonight, and to all of you who are also not interested in the holiday coming up, I get it. It's hard for me too.

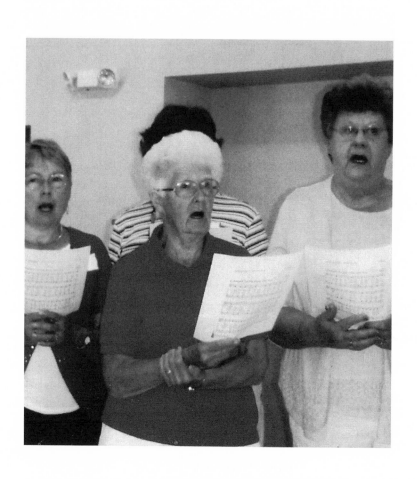

The Singer

It didn't take me long to find a picture of Mom singing. There were a few to choose from and I almost picked one with her wearing a sparkly-tree outfit, guiding the Sunday School choir. I'm not sure of the year of this one, but I would guess early nineties. It appears to be some special event, and I like that Mom looks healthy with her Maybelline Cool Watermelon lipstick and perfect hair. She must have just returned from Yuma, Arizona, because she looks tan.

Music has always been important to Mom. I love that she helped with the Bible School choir and Sunday School choir and sang in the Fron choir. She was a soprano, always in the front row, beside her friend Char. As a girl I waited for her on Wednesdays after school as they practiced in our church's high balcony. Even when she baked or made dinner, she hummed. It's a distinct memory for me.

A few months ago I visited Mom on a Wednesday, her church day. It's a nondenominational service and I know she enjoys going to it. I sat with her for a while and noticed she was softly singing. When the song ended, the pastor recited the service and Mom recited along with him. Word for word. I was surprised since I didn't even know or remember the words. Mom was always a devoted Lutheran and I loved the fact that she could still sing and remember the verses.

Music continues to be important to our family. Sophia made All District Choir this year as a fifth-grader and we hear her sing every day. She loves music as much as I do. Music, I believe, is good therapy.

Last month, Sophia and the All District Choir sang at Orchestra Hall. It was just beautiful. The high school then performed Handel's *Messiah*. I could almost hear my mom's voice singing to her favorite oratorio. Her own choir performed it a few times. I was thinking wistfully of how much my mom would have enjoyed watching Sophia sing.

Before her memory loss, Mom attended almost all of Sophia's preschool events, even going to a music class with her. She has missed a lot since those days, and it's not her fault. It's the disease that invades her and has taken her away from so many of our activities.

I was telling Sophia's music teacher how much we enjoyed the concert and how much my mom would have loved to attend, if she had been able. I shared a little about how much my mom enjoyed music and how proud she would have been of Sophia. And then you know what? Magic.

Barb and Beth organized the choir to come and sing for Mom and the other residents. I know it took a lot of work but they did it. My mom's sister attended, along with my neighbors Mary and Glenn (my Grandparents Day savior) and our family.

I wish you could have heard them sing. Mom was having a more alert day and I was trying not to tell her too much information. She gets confused quickly if I rush her, so I just said that Sophia was coming over to sing for her and she was bringing some friends. That seemed to get her interest. All of a sudden she was rushing and telling me to hurry.

Mom sat in the front and was a little cold and, at times, wanted her bed. But, overall, I could tell she loved it by her clapping and toe tapping. She asked her sister a few times where Sophia was. She was standing in the back and I think it was hard for Mom to see.

I wish you could also see the expression on Mom's face. Music erases memory loss; it really does. Other people were clapping, tapping, and loving it. It was such a beautiful thing to witness.

You know what else I loved? The kids weren't scared. Not one bit, as far as I could tell. It's hard to know what to expect when you witness something you're not familiar with. My girls have grown up with this disease and they are used to the loss and behavior that is not really their grandma.

They had cookies and hot chocolate afterward and we got to take a picture. I think I was more excited for them and how they made so many people happy for doing something so simple. I told people that Mom may not remember those forty-five minutes, but I sure won't forget how happy it made all of them. Huge thanks to all who were involved in this, especially Barb, Beth, Clare Bridge, all the surrounding schools for letting the kids out early, and the talented kids. You all made a difference and our family is grateful. So grateful.

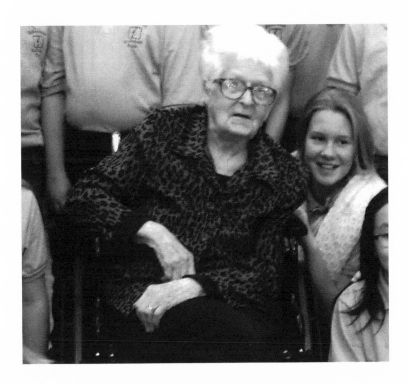

The Bed

It's been a while since I've been able to write or even have wanted to write. While there are some things that happen with Mom's care that I feel are appropriate to write about, there are others I don't. Many things stay private. Other things that occur seem to just flow into a story.

Over the last few weeks Mom has had some good days and some other days that I wish would move on into the next day. It's Christmastime, her favorite time of year, and I wonder if that's the cause of her worry. On my visits she's been asking the same questions, over and over again:

"Has Ross been here? Have I missed him?"
"I'm worried about Bud. Have you seen him?"
"You know I need to get back to Howard Lake. I'm late."

I answer that Ross, her son, is just fine and not to worry. Bud, her brother, is also fine. I remind her that I can call him and see if he can come over to see her. I let her know that I can take her to Howard Lake when it gets warmer, but it's currently too cold out. We have talked about her continued questions fifty times in the last few weeks.

This week I brought Mom to her room and tucked her in for a nap. She was tired and anxious and I felt I was not helping her much with her concerns. When I put her blanket over her, she asked if I would lie with her. I have been doing that lately since it seems to calm her. She moves over a little and I crawl in. I can hear her relax and she always grabs my hand.

I'm left listening to the building noise and her soft breathing and noting that she is sleeping. I can see her Christmas cards on the wall and I'm so grateful for the people who sent them. I can hear alarms going off in the distance and see one of the men, Melvin, pop in and ask if I've seen his daughter. I can see the birdhouse swinging outside her window and I know the birds wonder where I've been. I'm trying to relax beside her but my mind wanders in so many directions.

It has come full circle.

Earlier in the morning, Emme, my six-year-old, did the same thing. She had a bad dream and wanted me to crawl in with her. She is also nervous, scared, and wanting to be close to me. I end up letting her crawl into our bigger bed. How strange that this happens on the same day. Eighty-two years separate the two of them and both of them need my comfort. This is what a "sandwich generation" is all about.

It seems like yesterday that I crawled into bed with my own mom and dad. I remember their bedroom so vividly. The gold comforter sprawling over their twin beds pushed together. I can still smell the whiff of Charlie perfume, mingled with my dad's outfits and his smoke smell. I can still see the willow tree outside as it reached my parents' window with its limbs, making the softest noise, enough to make me think there was someone outside and scaring me all over again. I see my mom pulling back the covers and me cuddling with her warm body. To a young girl, that was heaven. It didn't happen often but enough for me to remember.

Now I'm in my mom's bed doing the same thing. I felt a little strange at first but I recognize that she also needs this warmth. She has her blue puppy on one side, and me on the other. Pray that we don't break her bed.

I was told yesterday that M died of a stroke this week. If you remember, she was the one who slapped my mom and was the only one who I told my kids to watch out for because she was so unpredictable. My heart was sad to hear of her death. This disease really touches so many. Who M was today was not reflective of who she was ten or even five years ago. She was a mother, daughter, and sister and I'm sure she had many friends who loved and supported her. And she taught my Emme a lot of language that she hadn't heard yet.

Feeding Mom tonight:

Mom: Should I know you?
Me: Yes, I'm Jodi, your daughter.
Mom: Do you live here?
Me: No, but I'm close to you.
Mom: There is room for you to sleep here.

Once a mom, always a mom.

The Four Men, January 2015

Today was my regular Thursday visit with Mom. Emme and I made blueberry muffins last night and I brought her bananas and caramel corn, which she loved. She ate almost everything and finished if off with coffee.

For the last month she has been asking about four different men. Today it was her father, Charlie. "Have you seen my dad today?" She has asked me this question before and it's the hardest question for me to answer. Her question about the other three men are easier for me for some reason.

In nursing school, you are told to be honest when a forgetful person asks you a question. I still find it easier to go with the flow and try to judge how your answer will affect the person. I've had many patients weep after I tell them their loved ones have passed away. Recently I visited a man right after his wife had died, which he had forgotten. It was like opening the wound all over again.

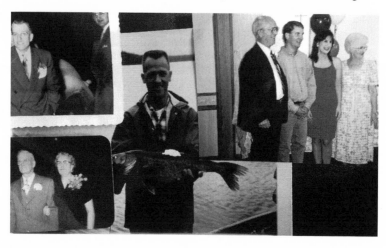

He had simply forgotten she had died. It was painful to watch his grief. Every day the aide reported that he would wake up and call for his wife. It's hard for people to imagine this and hard for me to witness it.

I find myself pausing, not knowing how to answer. Mom has asked me before and I told her that he is not here and she seemed all right with that. She seems to move on to either her brother, my brother, or my dad.

Today I told her that her dad has been gone for a long time, even before I was born. I told her that I've heard through family what a good father he was, raising four children and owning a country store. I can see the look on her face of sadness and she is quiet. I feel I should have told her he's not here, like I did before. I know she will ask about him again, just like she does about her mother.

She has been asking for these four men: Her father, her husband, her brother, and her son. All men important to her because they're family.

One, gone for a very long time and her memories of him must be surfacing.

One, married to her nearly sixty years and her love.

One, willing to come see her if we can get him a ride. Her connection to him still present after almost eighty-eight years.

One, having a difficult time with her loss.

All four men are coming up in her memories. I wish that heaven gave you five minutes with a loved one and that she could see two of them, knowing they are looking out for her from up above.

As I was driving home, I thought of a project I could do for her. I found pictures of each of them and will put them in a special frame. That way, when she asks about them, I will let her know they are right here, right beside her. I will put it by the picture of my dad. I hope this gives her comfort.

As I left today, she said, "You drive safe!" She is still my loving mother.

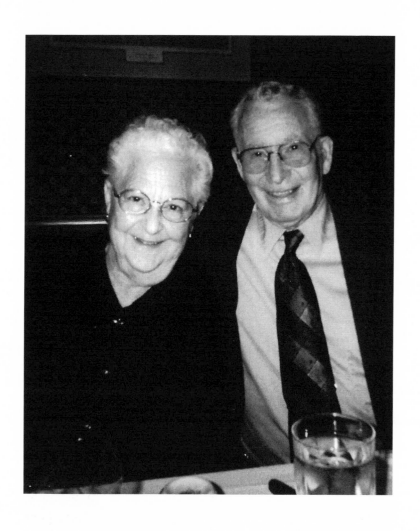

The Best Friend

My mom lost one of her best friends, Marilyn, and I have been sad all day. I love this picture of Marilyn and her husband, Don, so happy at our wedding. She has been a part of my life ever since I can remember, and I know my hometown is grieving her loss.

I think you are a lucky person when you find a human being you can connect with. My mom was lucky to have found Marilyn. There were many pictures to pick from, but I kept coming back to this one. I can still hear Marilyn's gentle laugh.

My first memories of Marilyn were driving in our old car heading out to Glacial Lakes State Park. She gave me a long lecture on my nail-biting habit, but softened the blow by saying that I had a "cute figure." I wasn't even sure what that meant at the time.

I used to spend hours at Don and Marilyn's house when Mom and Dad went out. We would go outside at night and watch the bats fly around, and Don told us they wouldn't bite us. I remember how their house was laid out and the hours we spent playing cards and how their kitchen table was a little nook. Marilyn was always baking and her kitchen always smelled of something delicious that she was most likely making for a church event.

After my dad died, Marilyn looked out for my mom and reported back to me. She was the one to call and say, "Your mom got turned around on her walk today," and "You know she is living off toast and cheese." She was firm, but gentle, and told me I needed to do something soon. Even though the words were hard to hear, I listened and did what she said. I moved Mom into Holly Ridge, and Marilyn was devoted to visiting her and taking her out to church and meals.

When I made the decision to move Mom closer to me, Marilyn was one of my first calls. I asked her opinion, and her advice was that Mom should live closer to me. She said we would both be happier. Again, she was correct. It was hard to move Mom away from her close friends, but I hoped they would see each other again someday. They never got the chance.

In the last few years I've received the sweetest, most encouraging cards and emails from Marilyn. She would remind me how much she missed Mom and tell me that I'm doing a good job of taking care of her and that she was proud of me. I have saved all of her cards and they hold a special place in my heart. Even though we were 120 miles away, I still felt her love. Just like a second mother.

Tomorrow I will bring her picture and let Mom know. We last sent Marilyn flowers a few months ago and I know Mom was happy about that. She knew that the name Marilyn was familiar to her. All those years of friendship.

Bless you, Marilyn. You were a loved friend.

The Bathtub

There are some days when I feel I'm doing a fairly good job with Mom's care, and there are days where I have no idea what the hell I am doing. I would say it's about fifty-fifty. Today, I'm in the latter category.

When we lived on our farm, Mom loved to take tub baths. Every Saturday night, Ross and I were forced to take a bath since church was the next day. We needed to be clean for the Lord.

Many times I would find my mom in the tub when I would come home from my activities at night. She had bubbles, a fresh towel beside her, and she would be reading a book. I think it was her quiet time from all of us. She'd wrap her hair in a towel so that she would not get it wet. God forbid that her salon-groomed hair would get wet in the tub.

Fast-forward to present. Since she moved into memory care she has not been able to bathe. They only have showers in the building. She has a wonderful bath aide through hospice and she gets a shower two times a week. I have helped the aide on many occasions and Mom complains the whole time. "I'm cold!"; "I hate this!"; "I need to get to bed!"; "Where is my baby?"

We finish as fast as we can and she is clean, smells wonderful of flowered lotion, and has new clothes on. I know she hates it, but I think she looks wonderful. I ask her if I can cut her fingernails and she not so politely says, "No, where is my bed?"

As I start to think about her showering at Clare Bridge, it dawns on me that we have a fairly large tub at home. I've given hundreds of people baths thoughout my nursing career. I could bring Mom to my house. I am almost giddy with happiness and can't believe I haven't thought of this before.

The next afternoon I pick up Mom in my car. It's getting harder to get her in my vehicle. I get a little help from Allen, one of the nurses. Mom has no idea what I have planned for her.

We drive the short way to my home. It's hard to see her so weak and tired, yet this does not deter me from my plan. The girls snuggle with their grandma and I make some coffee. We have ordered her favorite Chinese food and she eats more than I thought she would. Mom is flinching; she doesn't like loud noises or bangs, and I have told the girls to tone it down around Grandma.

While we are sitting together, I announce that I would love to give her a bath. She continues to sit there and not make a comment. "Mom, I brought you home to give you a bath. You haven't had a bath since you left Starbuck."

"Really?"

"Yes, really!"

I get up off the couch and enter our small bathroom. I gather some towels, my soft robe, slippers, and the bubble bath. I begin to run the water and I pour in the flowered-smelling bubble bath. I decide to light a candle and I start to feel giddy again.

I walk into our sunroom and she has already forgotten that I'm about to give her a bath. Sophia, Emme, and I pull her up out of the chair and walk the short distance to the bathroom. She is slightly winded and I can tell she is unsure of what we are about to do.

The girls want to help with the bath, but I tell them they can help once I get her in. I know that my mom has lost her modesty, but I want to keep her dignity intact with my girls and not have them remembering their naked grandma.

Emme is sullen that I won't let her help get Grandma in the tub. I help Mom use the toilet and I get her undressed. She keeps asking what I'm doing and I keep repeating that I'm going to give her a bath. Silence.

Her skin is wrinkled and dry. She is thinner than I have seen her before and she stands in all her glory hunched over. She looks at the tub and I wonder if she has forgotten what it is or how much it has meant to her over the years.

I notice right away that I don't have a bath mat for the tub and I'm mad that I didn't think of this detail before. I help her raise her left leg up to get it into the tub. She hunches over even more so and we are stuck until I can get her right leg over the tub. She starts to shake a little and I am starting to sweat. I realize, of course, that I need to get her to sit down in the tub and it is lower than I anticipated. I probably should have stopped then, but this was my brilliant idea.

I use motioning gestures to get her to sit down and she gives me a nervous look. I finally get her to kneel down and then I push her gently into a sitting position. I am totally full-blown sweating now. This was harder than I thought.

I can tell that her nervousness is starting to leave her face. She starts to play with the bubbles and I give her a washcloth to see if she can still remember to wash herself. She just slaps it on the water and doesn't use it as it sinks to the bottom. I will need that same washcloth later.

My happiness has returned. I remind her that she can put her legs down and that she can sink down a little bit more, like she has done for so many years. I am careful that she does not get her hair wet because I know that the beautician will be mad at me. I can see that her eyes are closed and I let her know that I will step out for bit while she relaxes. I close the door softly and yell to my family, "The bathroom is off limits for a while!" Sophia gives me a look and I remind her we have another bathroom.

I start to read for a few moments in my bedroom, enjoying a brief amount of silence. I get up to check on her and she tells me she is all right. I sit on the closed toilet next to the tub and enjoy this time, watching her relax. No memory loss in sight for the moment.

I ask her if she is ready to get out of the tub and she nods her head but doesn't move. I've got a towel on the floor outside the tub and I try to get her to stand up in the tub. One...two...three. Nothing. No movement at all. "All right, Mom. Can you help me, stand up in the tub?"

"No."

I'm not surprised and I'm not worried, at first. I have done this before for clients and I should be able to get my mother out of a tub. I try to show her how we get up with gestures but she gives me a blank look. I realize that there is nothing for her to hang on to, like the other places where I have worked.

I try numerous times to get her to understand what I am saying. I have taken off my pants to try to get her up, standing behind her and pulling up. I lift her and tell her to bend her knees and push off from the tub. "I can't! I can't!" I cannot believe the mess I am in. My mom is stuck in our tub and I can't get her out.

I tell Mom that I will be right back and I go in the sunroom to talk to Steve. "I can't get Mom out of the tub." He gives me a humorous look as he thinks I'm kidding him.

He gives me a look like only a husband can give when his wife asks him to help get his naked mother-in-law out of their bathtub. "I don't think I can." I tell him that I will try one more time and he agrees he will help me if I can't. I don't let the girls know what is going on because I think they would think it was funny. Someday I will also think this is funny.

Mom is still in the same position that I left her, but her eyes are closed and she tells me that she is cold. I'm sweating bullets and she is cold. I tell Mom that we are getting her out of this tub, come hell or high water.

I move her forward in the tub a little and plant a washcloth under her feet for her to step on for leverage. She and are I are both shaking a little. I step in the tub behind her, bend my knees and grab under her armpits and tell her to push up, knowing she has no idea what to do. With all my might, I heave her up to a semi-standing position. I gently lift her out of the tub with a strength that I had no idea I have. I've lifted my 120-pound mom out of our tub.

I grab a big bath towel and I wrap it around her tiny, shivering body and I wrap my arms around her and hug her for a long time. I can't believe I almost hurt her trying to give her a bath. I alert my husband that we made it out and I don't need his assistance. I'm not sure who is more grateful—Steve, who didn't have to see his mother-in-law naked, or me, that I didn't hurt her or my back.

When we arrive back at her memory care unit, I keep quiet about our mishap. I don't want anyone to think badly of me, though I did tell some close friends the story and they laughed, picturing my face.

I will never attempt a bath for her again, and I hope by the time she left our bathroom, she forgot our little adventure.

What kind of nurse am I?

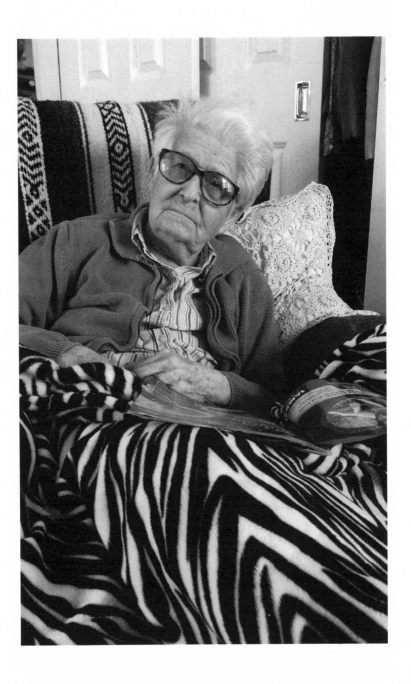

The Phone, February 2015

I arrive today to find Mom exercising (well, somewhat) in the courtyard. All the residents are in a circle and working hard with the activity person. I'm glad to see her out there; she is normally in her room or refuses to exercise. There she is in her black wheelchair, lifting her little arms and clapping when the staff person says to clap. I can hear her say, "I want to go to bed!" but still she continues the arm lifts. I laugh to myself, knowing those familiar words.

It's nice being able to watch her without her seeing me, although it's hard to watch her complete these simple, limited exercises knowing that in her past she was an exercise queen. Walked for miles, always moving and stretching in the morning. I should be glad that she is exercising. But I'm sad all the same.

Finally, she sees me and smiles. I smile, too, but I notice that she is not really looking at me. She is looking at what I am carrying. A huge bunch of bananas. I can hear her say, "Look at those bananas." Again, I start to laugh. She is pointing at them and she finally looks at my face and recognizes me. I feel like I'm not "The Girl," but I am "Banana Girl." She motions me over and tells me she wants to get to bed but she'd like a banana first. It's the start of a good morning for her.

When I get to her room, I'm reminded that I can't use her phone. I removed it a few weeks ago because I was worried she would fall when trying to answer it. There was also a man who kept calling her and I could not get him to stop. I wasn't sure if he was trying to scam Mom or if he just had the wrong number. He had a strong accent and I couldn't understand him well enough to find out why he kept calling. The decision to remove her phone was a hard one.

With the progression of this disease, I have had to stop or end many of her favorite things. Driving her van, balancing her checkbook, going for walks, cooking and baking. The list could go on but you get the picture. One of the last things she could do on her own was talk on the phone. Lately she had been answering the TV remote, and we had a laugh about that. There are such few things to laugh at, but we both found that funny.

I think of all the time I've spent on the phone with her. People comment on how close we are, the phone being an important factor in our closeness. I have called her for almost every important moment in my life: getting an A on my nursing paper, car problems, pregnancy updates, labor progression, heartbreak, money requests, updates about my dad. These phone calls were also the start of repetitive questions. She would call me and then five minutes later call me again with the same thing. The phone being our moderator.

When Mom moved into Holly Ridge in my hometown, I would set up her meds monthly and, instead of paying the cost of having the staff give her the meds, I would call her every morning and remind her. It was my time to connect with her and see how she was doing. It started to get hard when I was busy with my girls and work every morning and I would forget and panic. Plus, she would tell me she took them and I would find them still in the box.

When I moved her closer to me, I got her a phone. We could still communicate every day when I couldn't get up to see her. It was also my brother's way to communicate with her. I love how the girls would call Grandma and talk to her.

Over the past six months, it's been more difficult. Sometimes she would answer the phone and set it back down. I would need to call the front desk and have the staff hang up Mom's phone because she forgot about me or couldn't remember to press the off button. I thought long and hard about canceling it, and now I have. I don't think she knows it's gone, but I do. One more thing that has disappeared with this disease.

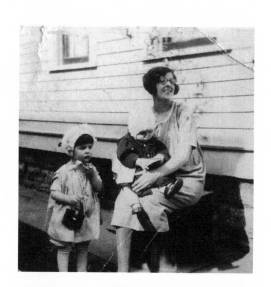

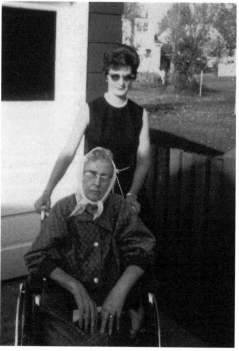

The Momma

This has been a long few weeks for Mom and me. We have both felt the good days and the bad days, and in the last few weeks she has started to call me Momma.

It started when she saw me and said, "Well, there's my Momma!" She continues to call me that when she sees me coming or watches me. I feel the term is a comfort to her and, in a way, endearing. There have been many names she has called me over the past few years. They include:

The Girl
The Flower Delivery Lady
Her
Gloria (her sister)
Jodi (on really, really good days)
And now, Momma

I went through her pictures today to show her what her own mother looked like. The first photo is from 1925 and shows my mom sitting on her mother's lap, along with her sister, Gloria. My grandmother had three children in three years and, as you can imagine, was very busy. The second picture is of Mom with her own ailing mother. Gloria, my aunt, has said they both took care of her until she died and that she was a good momma. I love both pictures.

Over the past few weeks, Mom has had a swollen hand and it has caused her discomfort. We had to take her ring off and she now holds her hand differently. Her palm was bruised up to her wrist. I'm not sure what happened. I hope someone just accidentally squeezed her hand too hard when getting her up. I worry about things like that. I have put her wedding ring in a safe spot and I may just keep it for now. She hasn't asked about it yet, but her hand looks different without it.

Last night, Steve dropped the girls off at church, so I spent some time with her. She was sick and threw up all over her bedding and pillows, all the while saying she was sorry. We cleaned her up and we watched TV until I had to pick up the girls. It's hard to see her sick. Again, she kept calling me Momma.

Last night was hard for me. Where do we find the most comfort when things go wrong? Our moms. I think she knows me as the person who comes to see her, brings her things, cuddles with her, and comforts her. To her, that is "Momma." I'm sure her mother did that for her, and she continued to do that with her own mother and with me. What a circle.

This morning I brought her new pillows and a banana. I found her at exercise class, but fast asleep in her chair. So very, very tired. She gave me a big smile and eyed the banana. She was pale and wanted to go to bed, so I transferred her into her chair and covered her up. While she sat in her chair, I asked her if she remembered my name. Easy as can be. Jodi. Not Momma.

Hospice continues. I've lost track of the days.

The Hospice End, March 2015

On Thursday of this week, I met with Cathy, our wonderful hospice nurse. I had been prepped last week that Mom would not qualify for hospice anymore. The rules have become much tighter regarding who can stay in the program; they must be actively dying. I understand but, to be honest, I'm happy and sad at the same time.

Actively dying is such a funny term. I think we are all actively dying to some extent. But some people are really truly dying. Mom has not lost any weight, has been feeding herself as of late, and just keeps holding her own. With the highs and lows of this year, I can hardly believe she is still here. She is a wonder.

For now I still get to see her, hold her hand, and just love her. That part of me is overjoyed. I know how rare it is to go off hospice. In all my years of nursing, I would guess I've had five people discharged from hospice. They just weren't ready to leave this world yet. I don't think anyone really wishes that a loved one will die. You may wish it for their sake but not for your own.

The hard part of Mom going off hospice is that she is still here. I can hear my dad somewhere yelling, "Shit, Jeanne. Hurry up and join me!" I know he's not-so-patiently waiting for her, along with all the friends she has lost. She sits in her chair and states every day that she wants to die. Every single day. I know it, I feel it, and I understand it.

It's not that I want her to go. I've spent all of these years with her and watched what an amazing life she has led. She will be eighty-nine in April and has graced this earth with all of her being. She's made an impact.

But, as a nurse and her daughter, it's hard for me to watch her. Slow, weak, disjointed at times, foggy, displaced, sad, overwhelmed with her life. She is not who she used to be and, even with her confusion, she is justified in wanting to die. I can't bring her back to where she was ten years ago. But I can be with her and peacefully get her to the end. It just isn't going to be right now.

There is hardly a week that goes by that I don't think of loss. Over the past two weeks, my mom's roommate has died. And my favorite Parkinson's patient had to put his beloved dog to sleep last week. This dog had been very important to him, fifteen years of love and companionship. We have watched the dog suffer over the last few months and it's been hard for him.

I sat with him the day before and he was struggling. He said, "I'm the only one who wants him to live; none of my family wants to keep him alive." I reminded him that not being able to get up anymore and being in pain isn't really living. The dog was helpful in getting him through sobriety and had a purpose. He was a very loved dog. I have heard before that we treat our pets much better than we do humans.

So on we go with the days, weeks, and months. The paperwork will return and I will continue my fight with Hennepin County and the hours spent figuring out her medical assistance and waiver status. Last Wednesday I was on the phone with the county for two hours, including hold time. The waiting drives me insane. I continue to call or email my friend Melanie about these issues. She is my hometown friend who is now an attorney in St. Paul and the smartest person I know. She answers my questions about Mom's care and billing that I can't understand. She is another part of my village that helps me with Mom.

Mom was officially on hospice for 171 days and continues to live.

The Weep

It's a beautiful day today and the girls and I decided to bring Grandma some Snickers bars and a few other things. We arrive and find her sleeping in her chair. The girls have never been known to be quiet and I think we woke her out of a deep sleep. She is disjointed and trying to tell me something, "That shouldn't happen!" I can't understand what she is trying to tell me, only that she is worried about something I can't figure out.

We give her a banana and she is worried that we don't have anything to eat and she keeps giving me the banana back. I tell her it's all right, that we just ate lunch. Again, I can tell she is worried and sad. The girls decide to read to her out of the devotion book. It normally is a comfort, but not today.

I try to help the staff when I can but the girls are with me and I know Mom needs to go to the bathroom. I help the kind older aide walk Mom to the bathroom and she keeps telling me, "Thank you, thank you." Both of us walk her back to bed and she starts to weep. I'm not sure if I hurt her walking or getting her into bed. She is afraid of something that she cannot articulate. I haven't seen her cry since September when she had her stroke and knew something was wrong with her. It's very difficult to see your mother cry, knowing that she is fearful of something. I again ask her a few questions and I can tell the aide is uncomfortable and does not know how to help. She has been weepy for most of the afternoon, he reports.

I decide to go get her some coffee, and I return to find my girls trying to help her. I think it is also hard for them to see Grandma cry. This is how I found them.

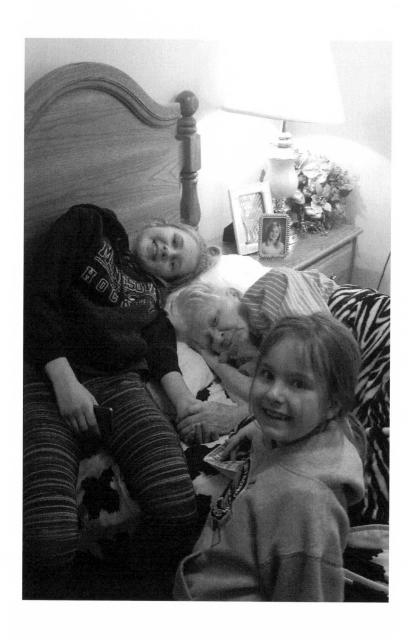

I love that they are trying to help and that she is holding Sophia's hand. She is calmer and less anxious. Over and over she says, "I love you. I love you. I love you."

I wish I knew what she wanted to say. Sometimes it's a guessing game and I get lucky. Sometimes she repeats what I've said. Today I wish I knew what her fear was and what made her cry. She is different in behavior today than she normally is.

I try to find the lesson. I know it's there. Should I be more patient? Can she see my own fear? What happens if she sees me cry? Today I'm not sure what the lesson is. Only that her fear and tears make me sad for her.

The Ambiguous Loss, April 2015

I want to share with you that these stories are hard to write. Really, really hard. It is a quick overview of our days, weeks, and months with this disease. Our roller coaster continues and this month has been no different. But, for some reason, this month has been harder.

I will share with you the good things first. My brother, Ross, came to visit her.

The week before he came I was feeding Mom lunch and she turned to me and said, "Is Ross all right?" I was surprised because it was totally out of the blue. I answered that he was fine. I didn't want to share with her that he was planning to come this weekend because I knew she wouldn't remember. I didn't want her disappointed if he couldn't come. She's been asking about him. He hasn't seen her for a while.

When he arrived, the first thing she asked was "Have you been lost?" I wish I could describe to you how alert she was, for which I was thankful. She was tracking well, funny, patting his leg, telling him that he needed to shave. Not once did she say that she wanted to die or that she had to get to bed, as she frequently tells me.

I was telling a friend that I think she must be bored with me. Every single day when I visit, I get the same two sentences: death and her bed. I am thankful that she was so alert for his visit. She has been asking about him again and I told her that he will come back and visit.

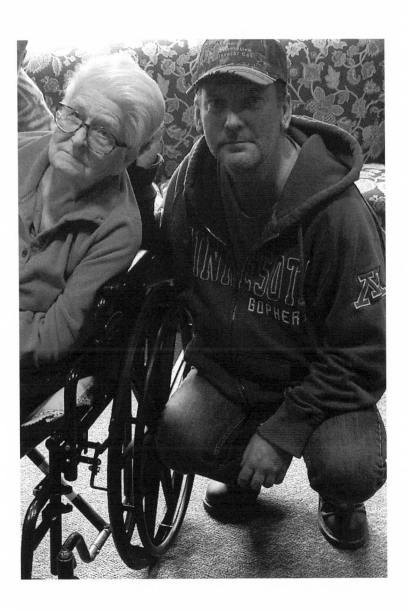

It is difficult with loss and grief. She is still our mother but not in the same way. Ambiguous loss is different from the loss through death because our closure is not possible yet and our grief cannot be resolved while she is still living. This loss complicates my own grief with her. The person we knew before is behind us and the person in front of us is now our mother. Funny, confused, kind, scared, coffee obsessed, and always loving.

She has fallen twice. The staff put her on the couch to get her out of the wheelchair for a while and they think she either fell off or got up to walk. The second time, she was trying to reach her Snickers from her bed and fell out. I had a message from the staff to move the Snickers. I am picturing her reaching for her favorite food and tipping right out of bed. She didn't get hurt, which I am grateful for. There is now a note on my counter to remind me to move the nearby candy, along with work notes and baseball reminders.

There is talk of her getting a hospital bed. I have mixed feelings about that.

Her Blue Dog is missing and she is mad at her baby and won't hold it. I don't know what to do.

Easter was not a good day for her. It's her favorite holiday and she was tired, leaning in her chair, and physically looked awful. The only funny part was when I told Mom that Steve, my husband, whom she has always adored, was here too and she looked at me and said, "Where did you find him?" Sometimes, she cracks us up.

Today she is sick. I fed her a little bit of lunch but she was not interested in food. She just said she wanted to die, and then she threw up. We put her to bed and she had the shakes. The aide, ever so attentive, and taking such good care of her. I asked her if she knew that her birthday was coming up and she said, "April 26." That should go under the good section. She is correct.

The Road Trip Home

It's a beautiful day today in Minneapolis. The brown grass is disappearing, the buds are blooming, and the sweet smell of flowers is in the air. Winter is over. Spring has arrived.

My mom's birthday is next weekend. I've been thinking what I can do for her. She will be eighty-nine years old, though today she denied she was going to be that old. I've been thinking about taking her for a car ride. She has not been out since the bath incident and I can hardly imagine being cooped up somewhere for the last few months, not being able to feel the outdoors or hear the birds sing.

Not getting her out has been hard for me. I have wanted to, but there have been many factors to consider. She hates being cold, her transfers are getting more difficult, and she is not the same as she was six months ago. I want her to smell the fresh air, see the beauty she has been missing, and see the places she has long called home.

"I want to go home!" "I want to go home!" "I want to go home!" She continues to tell me.

I know that to her, home is where she wants to be. As I have mentioned before, I'm not sure where home is. The red house in Crystal? The brick house by our own home in Plymouth? Her home in Starbuck or our farm? Or her home in Howard Lake? Home is where she wants to be.

I've decided to give her a road trip home. For obvious reasons I could not bring her to Starbuck or Howard Lake or even the place they lived in near downtown Minneapolis.

I wasn't sure if today would be a good day for her but, in all reality, every day is a tough day for her. I met her sister, her brother, and my cousin Bart at Clare Bridge. It was nice to see them and although she said she had to get to bed, I asked her if she wanted to go for a drive with us and she said, "Okay, that sounds nice."

So the following is our road trip today. I'd like to thank my co-pilot, Sophia, and Allen, who helped me with the transfer getting her into the car, which was a little tricky.

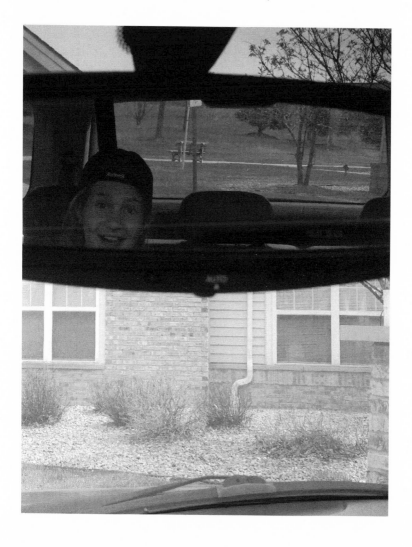

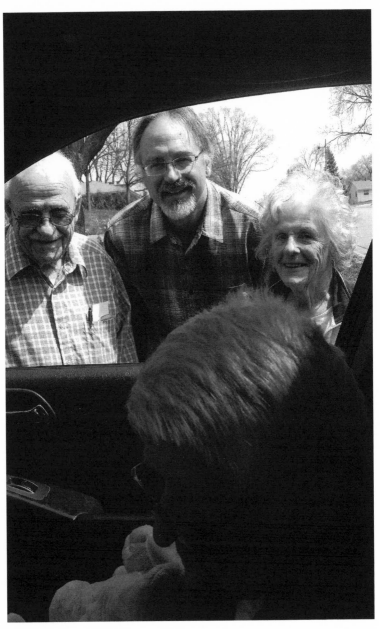

We stopped at her sister's house. Pictured is her sister Gloria, her brother
Bud, and my cousin Bart. Blue Dog came along for the ride.

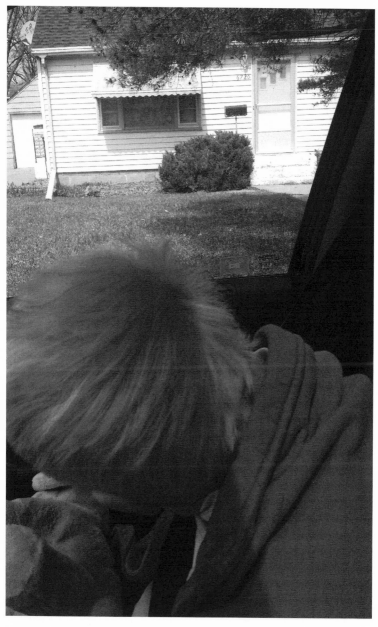

*This house in Crystal used to be painted red and Mom talks about this
house often. It's only a few blocks from her sister's house.*

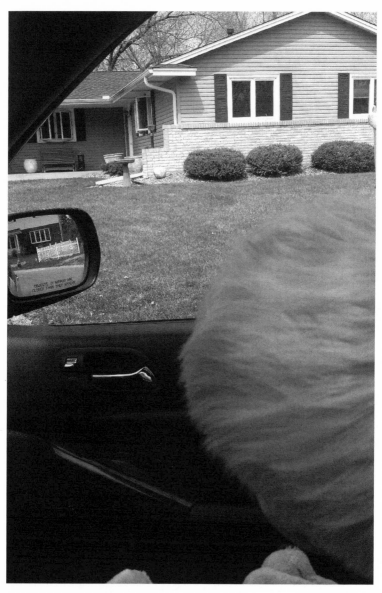

This is the house one block from our own house. The man who lived there was very gracious about letting us take a picture. This is the first house that Ross and I lived in when we were adopted. They built the house in 1964. Soon after, they moved to Starbuck, in 1970.

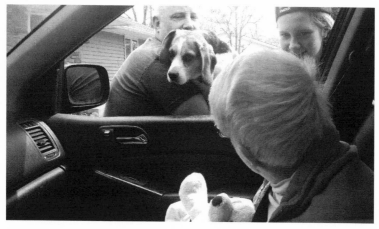

At our own home, where she visited us for many years. So many wonderful memories of time we spent together in our home. I felt so bad she could not physically get into our home.

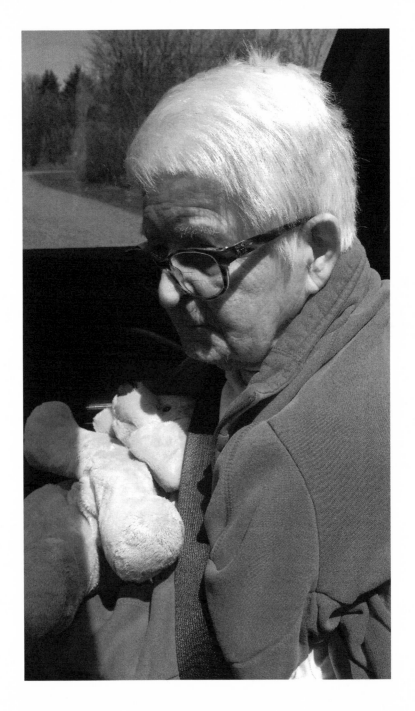

Part Three

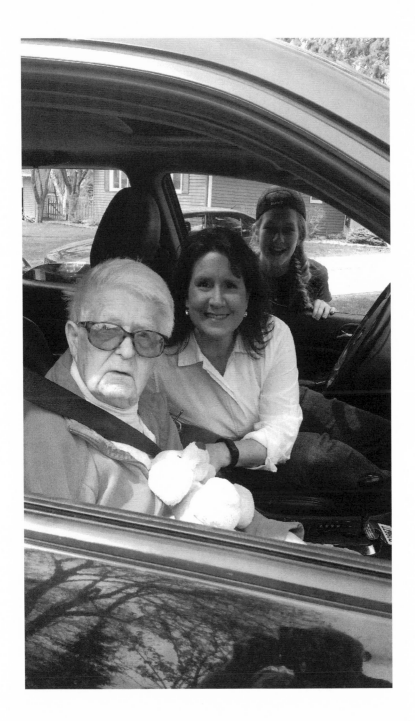

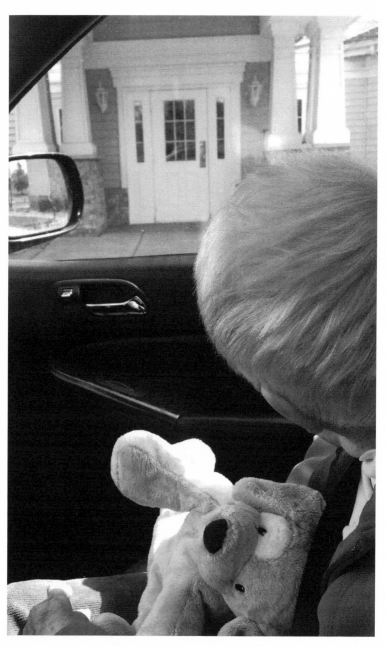

We arrived safe and sound. Blue Dog did pretty well too.

Driving back to her memory care, I kept thinking that this may be the last road trip we would take. The staff have asked if I am all right with her returning to hospice care again. She is not eating well, sleeps much of the day now, and is much quieter. I will call them this week and give my permission again. Round two with hospice care.

I know she won't remember today, but I will remember that we talked about her past homes and how she noted the color red of the Arby's sign. She commented that there are a bunch of blue cars and that she noticed the wind blowing against her face. If she can't ever get in the car again, I'm fine with that.

The Return of Hospice

Today, for two hours, I signed papers for the restart of hospice for Mom. She has been off hospice for two months and the nurses feel we should restart it. She is not eating very much, has had three falls in the last few weeks, is not verbalizing as much, and has lost a few pounds. Her spark is slowly fading.

I met the hospice intake nurse in a quiet back room and told her about Mom. Her name is Chris and she is gentle and kind. She has heard about Mom. I hope I am that understanding and gentle when I open my own nursing cases. We discuss massage and music therapy for Mom. We didn't use massage before and I want someone to professionally rub her back, like she always requests from me. We also requested to have Cathy again, Mom's primary hospice nurse.

On the first admission I was not emotional. It was something that needed to be done and I didn't have time to process the whole thing. Today when I arrive, I go to see Mom first and she is sound asleep on the bed and very pale. She doesn't respond to my voice. She is in such a deep, sound sleep.

I return to a small conference room to meet with Chris and start the paperwork. I'm listening to her but I can feel the warm tears start. I'm embarrassed that I start to cry in front of her but I have also watched the same thing with families on my own case opens. I'm not sure why, but for some reason today is different.

A few months ago, a woman I respect greatly told me it's all right to tell your mom that she can go. I completely understand what she is saying, but those are hard words for me to verbalize. For seven years, since my dad has been gone, I have taken care of her.

I have grocery-shopped in my small town, set up meds monthly, fought incorrect bills, paid bills, moved her twice, bought her clothes when she has lost weight, taken her on trips, yelled at people for her, and loved her. How do you tell someone you love that it's all right to stop living? But, like my client's dog, is this really living? I've thought about that conversation a lot.

When we finish with the paperwork, Chris and I return to Mom's room. She is in the same position. Curled up in a ball. She is wearing my old blue sweater that she loves. She has a huge hole in her nylons, crazy wild hair, and Blue Dog in her arms. Her baby is sitting in her wheelchair, just waiting to be held again. She refuses to open her eyes, even when I kneel down beside her. I introduce her to Chris and let her know what she is doing. Listening to her lungs, checking her feet, and looking at her swollen leg. In the middle of her assessment, still with her eyes closed, she says, "I think I love you."

We both start to laugh and I tell her, "I think I love you too!" She says she doesn't hurt anywhere and she is compliant and loving with Chris, repeating thank you, all with her eyes shut.

If I could show you what this disease is about or what it actually looks like, today would be the perfect day. The feeling of uncertainty, loss, and grief mixed in with a whole lot of love for a woman who doesn't want to open her eyes today.

As I was driving home, I was thinking about a book I read a few months ago about a woman with ALS. She wrote about the song in *Wicked* that describes her relationship with her daughter. It's called *For Good* and I thought of Mom:

"It well may be that we will never meet again, in this lifetime.
So let me say before we part
So much of me is made of what I learned from you.
You'll be with me. Like a handprint on my heart."

The Kiss, May 2015

In the past few days Mom has started to decline. She has been refusing medication, doesn't want to eat, and has been sick after meals. Her hospice nurse called me yesterday while I was at work, and we talked about adding or stopping medications and overall keeping her comfortable. Also, the nurse wants to start some morphine for her. I don't want to start it because I know where it leads, but it is a direction Mom desperately wants to go in.

After the call, I continue with my nursing visits, and then have baseball practice for the girls so I can't go see Mom right away. I was assured she was resting peacefully. I cry to a complete stranger at baseball when she asks if I'm all right. I cry at the stoplight with the thoughts of her dying. I continue to cry in the parking lot before I enter her memory care. I know the end is coming.

Last Thursday morning I had a dream about Mom. It was the kind of dream you have right when you are about to wake up. In the dream, Mom sat down by my side of the bed and kissed my left cheek a few times. I remember how vivid the dream was. She had gray hair instead of her stark white hair and she had her older glasses on. I could even see the numerous books on my nightstand. I felt like she was right in my room and I woke myself thinking, "How did she get in here?" I told Steve about the dream yesterday. It was so real. I felt I could reach out and touch her.

Today we have baseball for the girls and are trying to figure out our schedules. My priority is to see Mom. Emme, my six-year-old, has a gold heart on her dresser and I ask her if I could have it, just for today.

"No."

I tell her I was going to give it to Grandma today. Since I was giving it to Grandma, she was fine with that. "You can give it to Grandma!" So I gave Mom the gold heart and it sits by her bed.

I am so happy that in the past month she got to see my brother Ross, went for a car ride, felt the wind on her face, got a quick glimmer of "home," and celebrated her 89th birthday. I have enjoyed every minute I have spent with her and I know my dad is waiting. I am also grateful for the staff who take care of her with such love.

Before I leave, we sit in the warm sunshine on the patio. We can hear the birds sing, see the plants sprouting, and smell the fresh air of spring. She is asking for her momma and I tell her what a good mom she herself has been. She looks at me with one eye open and I know she heard me. What a good momma, indeed.

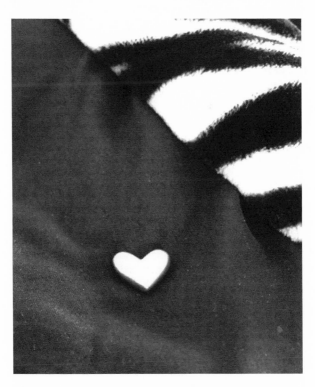

The End, May 2015

I am up early on this Saturday morning. I can hear the birds talking and can see the beautiful sky slowly waking up. I can't sleep. Sleep has been my enemy this past week. I am exhausted.

Early Wednesday morning, my mom left this world. At 4:20 a.m. to be exact. I'm now up and I feel she is shoving me out of bed. I feel she wants me to write but I'm not sure what she wants me to say. I will do my best.

For the past year, she has wanted to die. This is a fact she has repeated over and over. She has made this statement in the car, in her bed, on the toilet, watching the birds, and at meal time. Sometimes she looks at me to say, "Hey, I'm talking to you. Yes, you!" I've talked about this conflict a lot.

Last Wednesday she was not feeling good. She was sick at dinner, refusing her medications, and getting weaker. Cathy, her hospice nurse, talked about starting a little morphine for her, but I wanted to use Tylenol first. I don't think she has ever had morphine and I was worried it would sedate her too much, but I was still willing to try it when necessary. Saturday came and I was worried about her. We had discontinued her aspirin and I was concerned she had a small stroke since she was leaning so much. We couldn't get her to eat much and her head was tipped down so it made it hard to feed her. We were having a birthday party for her on Sunday since most of the family could not see her on her actual birthday. I called the family to update them.

On Sunday, we got her out of bed and put her in a tip-back chair so we could attempt to feed her. Most of her family came and we sat in the lovely courtyard with the birds flying overhead and the breeze on her face. She would wake up every once in a while, and I would tell her who was there. It was the last time she had her beloved coffee, only taking small sips. It was nice to spend this time with her, surrounded by all the people she loves.

On Monday, I knew it was serious. I found her in bed with my bright shirt on, hair neatly combed, and she looked like the bed could swallow her up. Her mouth was dry and we worked on getting small sips in her. Throughout the day, she kept trying to tell me something. I could tell she was frustrated I didn't understand her. At the end of the sentence, what came out clear was "I love you." A little garbled but I got it. Over and over again. I love you. I love you. I love you.

I had a special moment with one of Mom's aides, who told me that Mom was her favorite. She said that they didn't hit it off at first but they grew to love one another and spar back and forth. We had so many people checking on us.

My pastor, Beth, came to see her and gave her a blessing and anointed her. All those long conversations she and I had about my mom. That was a meaningful moment since Mom's faith has been important to her. I left about 9 p.m., telling her what was in my heart and not expecting her to be alive much longer. When I left, she just patted my left cheek, the same cheek that I had dreamed about her kissing last week.

When you are a nurse, you are the one to get the call that a client has died and it's so difficult making that call to let family know of their loved one's death. All night, I kept listening for the phone to ring. It didn't.

Tuesday, I got my kids to school and headed to Clare Bridge. When I arrived, Steve, the male volunteer, was holding her hand. He loved my mom and he came in early, before work, to say good-bye. I loved that he still called her Mean Jeanne. It was a very touching moment.

Mom was now not able to talk. The voice that I've heard my

whole life is now gone. We had started a small amount of morphine to keep her comfortable. When I would say the word "Mom," her eyes would flutter. What an important word for her. Mom.

It's hard to express how kind people were but I'm not surprised. We had a busy day of people coming and going. The nurse, the social worker, massage therapist, music therapist, and two pastors, who again blessed and anointed her. I love that she was blessed twice. The room smelled of oil and lavender. I swear to you, a bird came to the window and kept knocking at us throughout the whole day, as if to say, "Hey, I'll fly with you when you are ready."

When I left on Tuesday night, I was exhausted. My enemy, sleep, was winning. I had fallen asleep twice in her chair and tried to lie by her side but the bed was too small. They traded out her normal bed for the hospital bed. After all those months of crawling in with her, I could now only sit by her on the bed.

When I left her, I was aware of something important. I knew that she wanted to die without me there. I knew that in my heart. I told her she could go and that her job here on earth was done.

My phone rang at 4:20 a.m. and she was gone. Her soul finally at peace.

As you go about your days and weeks, remember my mom when you see or smell the following things:

- Lilacs. We had them on the farm and she loved to put them in a pretty vase.

- Fresh-brewed coffee. Black, nothing added, as it should be.

- A Snickers bar.

- A rhubarb plant or stalks. I will continue to make her rhubarb recipes.

- A child's laugh. She loved kids to the moon and back.

- A Dairy Queen. Boy, did she love our hometown DQ. A small cone or a Snickers Blizzard.

- Lemon bars. I made her recipe yesterday and it filled the house with her memory.

- A choir singing. Picture her humming along.

- Any kind of book. She taught me that the best escape is with a book.

Finally, do some random act of kindness. She was all about helping her family and friends. Thank you for all of your sweet messages. I can read only a few at a time. Your words are important in getting me through. One of my friends said, "You loved her well." I love that. We both loved each other well.

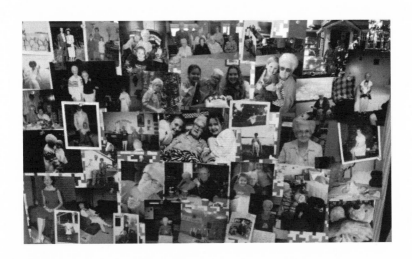

PART FOUR

Carry On

The Grief and the Gratitude,
June 2015

"Perhaps they are not stars in the sky but rather openings where the love of our lost ones shines down to let us know they are happy."
—Eskimo proverb

I'm up early again. The breeze is coming through the window. Barley, our beagle, has had his treat and everyone is still sleeping. It's a quiet time for me to write. It's been thirty days that my mom has been gone. One full month. The void of her has been hard.

Grief is a tricky thing. Just when I think I'm doing all right, I see or hear something that triggers a memory. It ebbs and flows through me and it feels to be almost constant right now.

Grief seems to be all around, with friends also experiencing this shadow of pain. I have friends with a new loss of their dad and sister. I have a friend who lost their family home. I have friends in the hospital and client families trying to work through their own grief over their loved one. Grief does not discriminate.

Yesterday, I was at an assisted-living building completing a medication change. I wanted to get in quickly and leave. But when I was entering the building, I stopped to watch a daughter trying to get her mother in the car. I watched for a while because I noticed she was having a hard time getting her in. I noticed the loving care she was providing and my own thoughts went to my mom's car ride, only six short weeks ago. I completed the medication change and was teary in my car. I miss the simple act of getting her in the car.

I think part of my grief ties in with gratitude. I have been overwhelmed with kindness from my family, friends, neighbors, strangers. Who knew my eighty-nine-year-old mother touched so many lives? I wish my mom could have known the generosity of people in the past month. Since her death, I could not begin to tell you how many people have helped. It was almost like a revolving door at our house with people bringing over food. Really, really good food. My eleven-year-old daughter, Sophia, told me, "So when people die, you bring people food? I hope this never ends!"

I have received food baskets in the mail, along with chocolate-dipped strawberries. I received a book in the mail from my friend Lisa in California that was called *H is for Hawk*, about death and hawks. (I cried like a baby when I got it.) I have received beautiful wind chimes that play a soft melody in the breeze. My work gave me a beautiful stone that I can put in my garden, along with time off and loads of food. My friend Joanie drove all the way to St. Cloud to deliver dresses to us the day of the wake because we had forgotten them in our garage. Joanie is also the person who found the same Blue Dog on Amazon when Mom's original one went missing a few months ago. Somehow, she found the same dog and ordered two of them so if we lost another one, we would have an extra.

And the cards we have received. I have finally read all of them, and I am still getting them in the mail. I hope you realize it will take me one year to thank you all. Emme counted them as a project; there are over 400 people to thank.

There are times in the grief and gratitude that I feel her around me. For the first week she was gone, I kept waking up at 4:20 a.m., the time she passed away. I'm not sure if it was conscious or not, but it started to be annoying. Plus, those who know me well know I'm not an early bird.

A couple of days after her passing, I had to run to Macy's to get a new shirt for Steve. The sweetest woman helped me, as I was in a hurry to get other things done. We found a shirt quickly and when we got to the register there was a line. She let me in first, explaining to the line that she had been helping me and it would take a minute.

In line, there was an older woman. Hair perfectly done, Burberry rain jacket, and a cloud of perfume. She was angry and said, "Well, we really don't have a choice, do we." I was quiet for a while, now feeling bad that the Macy's person helped me first. I softly said, "I'm sorry, my mom just passed away and we are heading out of town." Her response was, "Well, that's too bad!" still in an angry voice.

By this time, I'm upset. What I really wanted to say to her was almost out of my mouth. Really bad things that are not my normal. But, for some reason, other words popped into my head. Take the high road. It was my mother telling me that it's all right; not everyone is kind and understanding. I walked away, taking the high road.

I also feel her around me when I watch the birds at her bird feeder. We put the feeder in my garden, right outside our sunroom. I have been watching the birds joyfully feeding on the bird food and think of my mom watching her own birds at the memory care unit. Birds have become more meaningful for me, especially after that one bird knocked on Mom's window waiting to fly with her. Hospice sent me a beautiful card this week, with all the staff signing it. Kind and special words spoken about my mom and me.

For the last few years, Mom had a difficult time remembering my birthday. She would always ask, and a few times I could tell she was writing it down. While putting away some pictures, I found this.

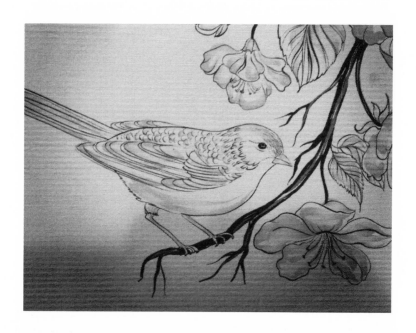

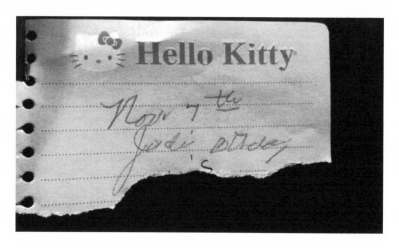

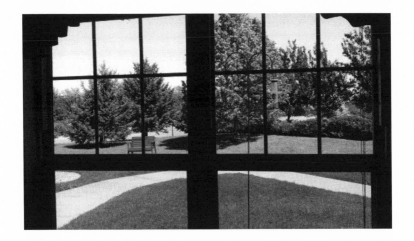

I know she is around me. Gosh, I miss her love. I hope she knows that both Blue Dogs are very loved and that I made her rhubarb dessert this week. I hope she knows that Sophia got a special award at school this week and Emme made it to second grade. I hope she knows that I drive past Clare Bridge every week, because we have two clients near there, and it's hard to know she isn't there anymore. The hardest day for me was cleaning out her room. I took this last picture, where you can see the view she had for almost three years. The bird feeder is visible, along with the bench we frequently sat on and talked about life.

The days, weeks and months will continue and I know she is where she wants to be. Grief and gratitude will continue but hopefully one of them fades away.

The Gifts and the Signs, July 2015

For the past several weeks, I have continued to receive thoughtful gifts from friends. It's been two months, and life continues to move on. I was talking with my friend Leanne and we both agreed that receiving cards and gifts months after your loved one has gone is wonderful. Don't worry about being late with cards or gifts. Everyone is busy. Just to know that people care is what's important.

Here are just a few gifts that have touched my heart in the past few weeks.

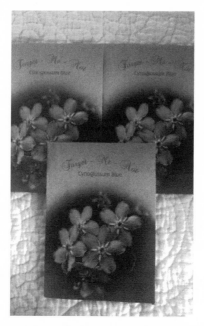

My friend Rich sent me forget-me-not seeds, which are significant within the Alzheimer's Association. Rich, you are a gem and the kindest person I know.

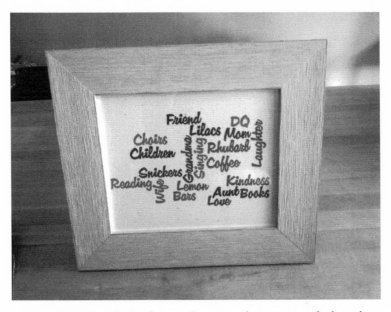

My friend Anne made this for me. She captured my mom perfectly and it sits by her picture. I LOVE it. You are the best, Anne.

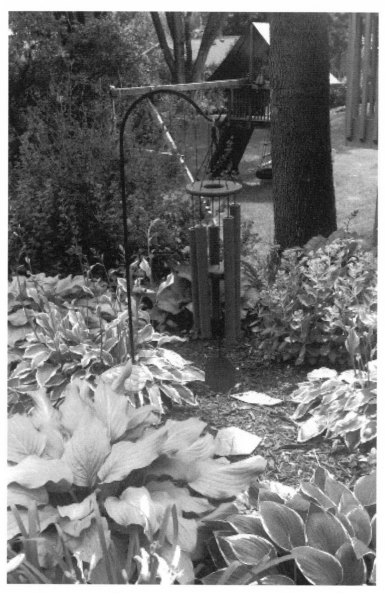

Our friends Jim and Cristy sent me chimes. I love how they fit into my garden, close to Mom's bird feeder. When a storm blew in last week, I could hear the beautiful music in the middle of the night. They also sent me a lovely card that is displayed on my desk.

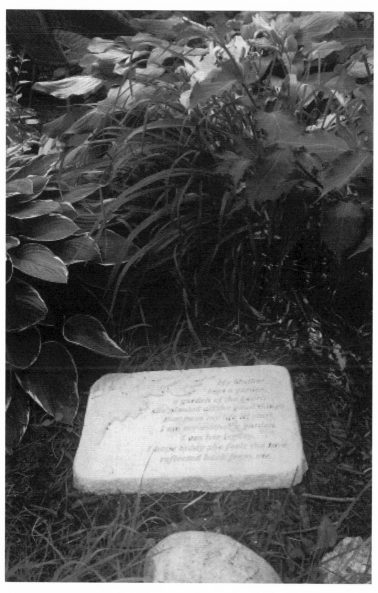

My stone marker from my co-workers sits right by Mom's bird feeder. It's incredibly special and I love that bird seed spills out on it. Mom would have loved this. I'm blessed to have a great nursing family and community.

I think that when anyone loses a loved one, it's normal to look for signs. I feel Mom around me in subtle ways. When I was assessing a client at a rehab facility in Bloomington, there was a storm warning. Staff needed to move all the residents into the hallway to keep them from being scared. The activity aide started to play her guitar. The first song she played was "Edelweiss" from *The Sound of Music*. This was one of my mom's favorite songs, and when Mom was dying the music therapist played this for her on the guitar. I recorded it, hoping she would sing along. She didn't sing, but she did listen. She always loved music.

One of the other signs is her bird feeder, sitting in our garden, right outside our sunroom. There is a yellow finch that comes often. I'm sure it isn't the same bird that visited my mom's room the day she was dying, but I'd like to think so. Steve says it is a male because of the bright colors. The finch comes and goes while I have been watching him, just like my mom watched the birds while in her memory care unit.

It's hard not to think about her. I still get mail for her almost every day. I'm working on finishing the thank-you cards and trying to figure out how to honor Mom with the money people have sent me. I think about getting a bench in her memory or maybe giving away Dairy Queen treats.

The feeling of grief is still there. I sometimes wonder if I should be so sad about a woman who was ready to die at eighty-nine, especially when I think about a mother who has suddenly lost her young child or a woman who lost her sister or a man who lost his dog, all sudden and unexpected. I was prepared for Mom's death but I still feel unprepared for the void she leaves. My friend and neighbor Mary reminds me that I was with my mom for forty-five years and that some people don't get to experience their loved one for that long. She is correct.

We all feel grief and we all are tied together by loss. It doesn't matter what the loss is. Loss is loss.

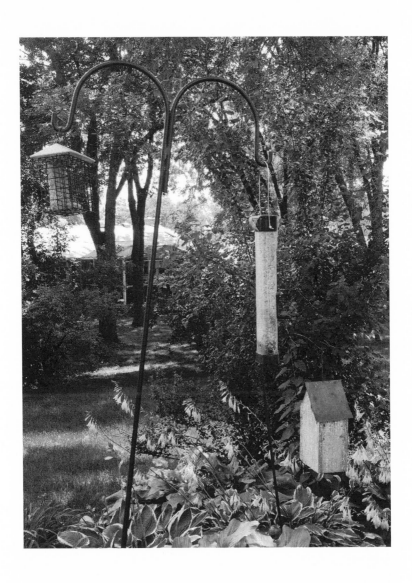

I hope the signs continue.

Blue Dog

Emme has been full of questions lately. I know she has been missing Grandma, as we all have. Here are some of her questions:

- How do you become a grandma?

- Once you are a grandma, do you stay a grandma for your whole life?

- Do you think Grandma can see me from where she is?

- When do I become a grandma? (That was tonight.)

This whole week I have tried my best to explain the term *grandma* to her. I even told her that I had an adopted grandma named Julia growing up because one of my grandmas died before I was born and the other one died when I was young. We adopted Grandma Julia Danielson and we showed Emme pictures of her. She knows that I am adopted and we talked about Grandma not being able to have children and why. I think her brain was on overload today.

Today she again asked if Grandma watches over her. We have talked about heaven and our beliefs, but I feel like she looks at me and wonders if I'm telling her the truth. In the past few weeks she has asked if Grandma lives above the moon. She has also asked if she lives on or above the clouds. People have told her that Grandma lives in her heart. How can she live in her heart?

Today we talked about Blue Dog, my mom's stuffed animal. I thought about this a lot today and I told her that I think Blue Dog

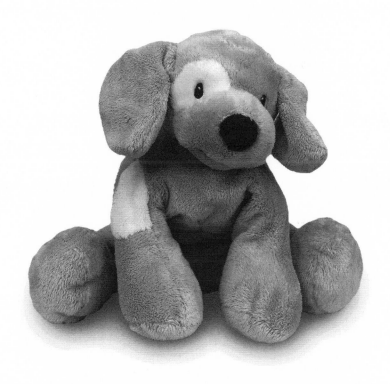

is here to watch over her for Grandma. I reminded her how much Blue Dog brought Grandma comfort. This seemed to make sense to her. Guess where Blue Dog has been today?

- It went down the slide with her many, many times today.

- He (I think it's a he) ate cereal with her in bed.

- He went in the car with her but I wouldn't let her bring it in to Perkins.

- It's been in the baby stroller, watching the kids play.

- He took a badly needed nap this afternoon

- He wrestled with her, along with her dad.

I hope that I'm not confusing her. As a parent, I wonder what to tell her. I miss her grandma too.

To be seven again and wonder what this world is all about. Blue Dog is in for some adventures, along with her favorite animal, Lambie.

The Parentless Daughter,
September 2015

A few weeks ago, we buried both of my parents. The heat index that day was way over 100 degrees, but I know that my parents would have loved the beautiful day. There were boats on the lake, pretty flags flying in my hometown, and the Dairy Queen bustling with people. It was a perfect summer day and a special day to honor my parents.

At age forty-five, I feel a bit lost with both of my parents gone. When they adopted my brother and me, they were older parents already. They were both forty-three when I was adopted, twenty years older than the parents of my friends. I've always known how much they wanted children. I think they adapted well to being "older parents."

My brother and I were lucky to have them for as long as we did. My dad died at age eighty-one and my mom lived two weeks past her eighty-ninth birthday. That's a long time to be loved by them. We were both lucky to find one another and bridge the gap.

I have lived many adult years but I will always be a child in relation to my parents. Even though I took care of both parents before their deaths, they were still the parents of my youth that I buried. I think the world is a different place after our parents die.

My relationship with my parents wasn't perfect. Few of us have trouble-free relationships with our parents. Some of us look back and remember harsh words spoken and other problems. But we should know that our parents forgive us, and we need to move on.

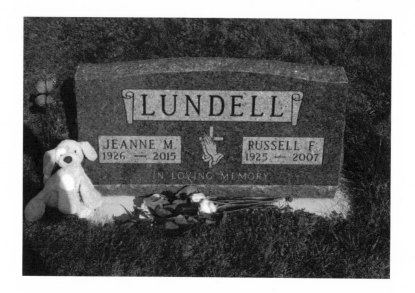

Nothing will ever be the same after losing my parents. Mom and Dad will not be there to applaud my accomplishments or give me direction at an important crossroad. They won't be able to see Sophia do well in school or watch Emme sing in the choir. They will miss many of our life events.

I will treasure all the memories from my childhood and adulthood that they gave me. All those lessons they tried to teach me. Some successful, some not so much, like sewing and making jam. We are who we are because of their love and nurture. They have guided me as best as they were able.

For all of you who have lost a parent or both parents, hang in there. Sorrow is deep and real. Talking to my family and friends has been helpful. Grief is present but not overbearing.

For those of you who still have your parents, enjoy them. I love seeing all the grandparents at hockey and baseball games and seeing all the parents of my friends. Our parents are a gift that lasts only so long. Ask questions about their lives. Be involved in their care (if able). Remember that we are all getting older. Don't let pride stand in the way of a past issue. I had a client's family tell me today that the time with their mom, who is dying from breast cancer, was not enough. They reminded me of myself four months ago. Life is short.

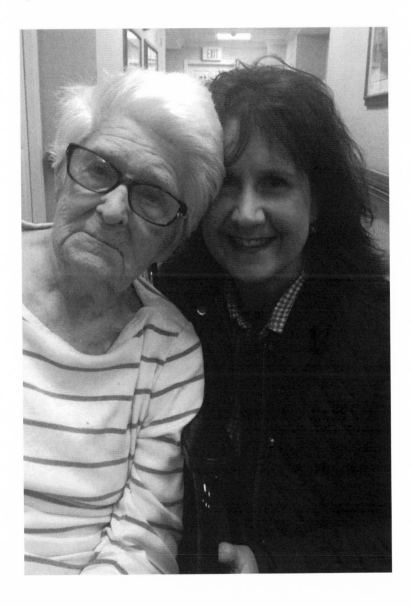

Six Months, November 2015

It's hard to believe that Mom has been gone for six months. There is not one day that I don't think of her or that I am not reminded of her or my father. I feel like I've been given little reminders of both of them in the last six months.

On the seventh of this month, I celebrated another birthday. Over the past few years, I have celebrated with Mom at her memory care unit. I would remind her that it's my birthday and she would become sad because she forgot, and I would try to make her happy with cupcakes, Snickers, and coffee. The day before my birthday was the six-month anniversary of her death. Boy, I miss her voice. The picture on the previous page was from my birthday last year, November 7, 2014.

When I was at the grocery store this week, I brought a bunch of change to put in the coin exchange machine. Sitting right next to the machine was a woman in her late eighties. She sat on the bench with her legs crossed, perfect hair, a rain jacket on, and small bags of groceries at her feet. I noticed how tiny she was as she sat very quietly with her hands crossed in her lap.

She gave me the sweetest, kindest smile. As you can imagine, she reminded me of Mom. She watched me pour the change in and she asked me a few questions. Simple talk. She was my mom probably seven years ago. Interested, kind, alert. I so badly wanted to sit down with her, hug her, and tell her how much she reminded me of Mom. I also thought she probably thinks I'm a nut. I got in my car and thought she was a little sign from Mom. I'm also proud that I didn't cry when I was talking with her.

Do you remember that bird that kept tapping on Mom's window when she was dying? I still have her bird feeder in our backyard, right outside our sunroom. I ran out of bird food and bought some new food for them. Guess what? No birds. I even moved the feeder to a tree in our front yard. Steve thought they didn't like the food, so I went to the store again and bought new food. Again, no birds. I have moved the feeder to different spots and this week I noticed a cardinal sitting on top of the feeder, not eating, just staring at me. I think the birds have flown away for the winter or I hope they are off flying with Mom somewhere.

I haven't been able to let go of her clothes yet. It seems so silly not getting rid of them. They are just sitting in buckets waiting for someone to use them. I was talking with my friend Carrie at hockey about her mom and I asked her if she needed any clothes. She said yes and I realized that my mom would want her clothes used by someone who needs them. I will keep some of my favorite items, but I realize after six months that I can let go of her clothes.

Grief is ever present but has lessened. It helps me to see my aunt Gloria, my mom's sister, who is just a miniature version of my mom. Emme interviewed her for a school project; I love that my girls still have someone to talk to. Many of you have lost parents, grandparents, friends, and loved ones. The loss is incredibly hard. I have a hard time when people say to remember the good times. I do remember the good times. But I would much rather talk to her or hold her hand again. Just one more time.

Over the past six months my mom has missed the start of school and hockey for the girls. She has missed Emme getting a special award from school and Sophia almost getting straight A's in her first year of middle school, with the exception of a B in shop tech! (My dad is laughing somewhere!)

She has missed my recent attempts at cooking, some winners, some losers. I'm trying to cook and bake more. (Somewhere Mom is laughing!) She has missed the frustration I sometimes have over things I cannot control. She always said, "Let go and let God."

She has missed how hard Steve works and how much the girls adore him. He is coaching them in hockey and he helps the girls in math, since I can't understand the new math. She has missed a lot, but somewhere, somehow, she knows. And I hope she knows how much I love and miss her.

The First Year, May 2016

I have stopped and started this entry many, many times. It's hard to sum up the first year without Mom, and over the past few days I've thought about what to share with the people who read it. May 6 marked the first year without my mom.

I have missed her.

Sometimes I think to myself, Why should I be so sad that she is gone? It's not like she wasn't ready to have her life end. She wasn't my young daughter who has her whole life in front of her or someone's brother who lost his life early to cancer. She was eighty-nine years old with a horrific disease that plagued her ability to eat, walk, show emotions, make her own meals, or even recognize me. I'm sure she's happy to be free.

I still miss her.

The first few months after her death I was filled with an overwhelming sense of love from people. People are so kind and loving. People ask how I am and they have certainly lifted my spirits. I grieved but I would call it a healthy grief.

The holidays were hard. She loved the holidays and it was different not to have her around. People talk about losing a loved one and the finality of it all. Holidays are tough.

I miss her voice.

Books and specialists talk about what stress and grief does to you. My grief came out in my hair. My hair literally changed after Mom died. The texture and shape changed—it became kinky and straggly and I looked awful. I can barely stand the pictures of me. It was almost like whatever was inside of me was coming out via my hair. I had my thyroid checked and my friend Martina, who cuts my hair, kept stating that she sees this with people who grieve. I spent a lot on hair products with no results. Awful, dull, lifeless hair. And that is how I felt.

I miss her love.

January was a very tough month for me. I felt like something had come over me and that I was an angry person. I was anxious, yelled at my husband and girls, yelled at people at work, and could not overcome what was wrong with me. I wasn't even reading. I could barely stand to look at myself. Grief.

I miss every stage with her.

There are stages of grief that anyone goes through and I'm sure I've hit them all. You miss the days of being a little girl and having your mom show you how to ride a bike. She introduces you to the world of reading. She teaches you how to be kind to the kid on the bus you want to smack. She teaches you to stand up straight. She teaches you that friends are important. She teaches you that neat handwriting counts.

You miss the high school and college years when she teaches you to be independent and watches you become a nurse. She is so excited for you and she watches you meet a boy named Steve and get married. You have two cute girls that are named after her.

You miss the days when your roles are reversed and you must take care of her. You gladly pay her bills on Wednesdays and visit her after work and on weekends. You introduce the world of Alzheimer's disease to your daughters and they love her all the same. You watch a beautiful woman ask her own daughter if she is indeed Jodi. You watch the kindest woman slowly slip away.

You miss all the stages that you have been through with your mother.

On Mother's Day, my second year without her, I spent the day with my girls and their numerous adventures. I stayed off social media with the exception of posting a picture of my girls enjoying ice cream at a favorite stop. I had butter pecan, my mom's favorite. (After a Snickers Blizzard, of course!)

I miss her smacks.

In honor of her birthday, on April 26, we donated Snickers Blizzards and cones at her hometown Dairy Queen. Thank you, Carrie, for helping me. I love the idea that we celebrated with her favorite treat. I hope she was proud of the way we celebrated it. I know we loved doing it.

I miss her when I see clients who remind me of her. Families ask questions and, on a rare occasion, I will tell them about Mom and her journey with the disease. Families also ask about the dying process and I share what may be to come. A few weekends ago, a woman thanked me for explaining the death process to her after she made the decision to come see her dad. It was the same way with Mom.

I think about her when I see a cardinal, smell our lilacs in the backyard, make her rhubarb torte, and see Emme snuggle with Blue Dog.

I miss just being her daughter.

The very first year is over with, and I'm feeling better. My hair is back to normal. My heart isn't so angry and I feel back to what is semi-normal. I'm not sure what more I can tell you about us. Just that I gave my best and loved her hard, and I'm proud that she picked me and that she was my mother.

The Journals

Over the past few months, I've had a chance to read my mom's beloved journals. As I've been organizing her bins, I've found a few more of her calendars and her journals that she was so dedicated to. They are a treasure. I know she has many more, but in her numerous moves over her life, some have surely gone missing. But I'm thankful for the ones I do have.

My mom actually wrote about how often my brother and I called her. Really. She even commented when she didn't hear from us and wondered what we were doing and why we hadn't called.

Many of her writings start with calendars. Then her trips, her meetings with Lutheran Social Services, and her views of her day with both Ross and me. I love that she documents her struggle with adoption and joy by writing in that tiny little space.

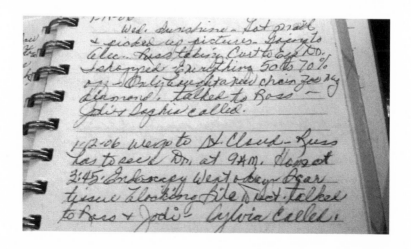

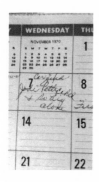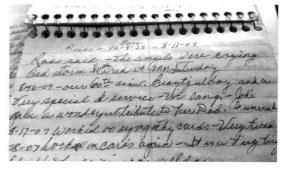

She writes about the weather, her walks every morning, my dad's golf outings, who she saw on her trip to the mailbox, who has died in the community, the birth of both of our girls, the sadness regarding my dad's death.

She writes about her close friends, baking buns and lemon bars for funeral services, and trips that we took after my dad died. She talks about her much-loved Dairy Queen in my hometown and her many years of cleaning houses after she retired from cooking for seniors. She writes about all the blankets she made by hand. She is grateful. Many of the entries are of her faith and her love for us. I love that in one of the entries she says, "Thank you, God."

Her journals are a snapshot of the start of her memory loss, achingly spelled out for me to read. She writes about her forgetting the eggs in the brownies and there is a confusing entry of her and the van. I think she got turned around somehow. She talks a lot about being tired and "getting mixed up."

I remember wanting her to have an MRI of her brain, and she agreed after much coaxing. I was having a hard time with the start of her loss, half in denial, half knowing that she needed more help.

As I continue reading, it becomes more difficult. It's the start of her memory loss in 2007. Her notes and entries start to get shorter and her handwriting starts to change. Her last green journal is filled with a quick synopsis of her shortened days. She

7-11-08 Fri-

7-12-08 - Luther Crest Bible camp quilt auction — I didn't go.

7-13-08 Emma Marie Nelsons — born 2 am. Brown hair — 7# - 1 oz. 20" long. — church— Church in the evening outside — went to bank

7-14-08 Pat organized to go to Jodis on Tuesday

7-15-08 Drove to Jodis — Got there just before they got home with Emma. What a sweet little girl.

7-16-08 Wendy to see baby in afternoon

8-21-08 Nice + cool — no humidity Walked - Washed clothes. Beautiful day made C.C. dish made buns + talked to Jodi + Ben Thank you, God.

8-22-03 Nice cool morning Walked Clean for Audrey. A + W for supper

8-23-03 - Walked — nice cool in A.M. Washed bedding - Have cleaned Windows + Blinds + curtains

930-07 - Choir practice. Helen Claire & ...
were Greeters - Rained hard - But when
church was out. I didn't accomplish
much today - Wrote some notes.

10-1-07 Had MRI of my head in Morris -
Carol came to Hosp- at 11 and waited for me
It was quite an experience - We ate lunch
at Pizza Hut.

2011
2-25 Exercise
2-26
2-27 - Church - Lunch at noon Waters Edge.
2-28 Went down to deer help with Crossword puzzle
spilt my coffee on puzzle.
3-13 communion 9:30 - Sunday
30
3-26 - Shaw Bthday - Jodi, Steve, Stephan & Emma here
to dinner at Edge - Ross, Heather, her mom - all to
Edge for dinner. Very nice - Jodi & Emma busy
around here.

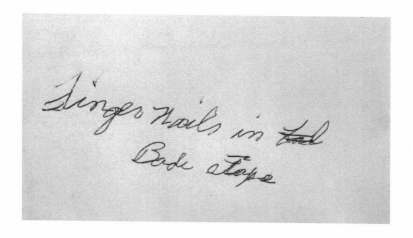

wrote only a short amount after I moved her into assisted living. I know she wasn't happy with me. She stops writing. This was her last entry.

I love that her last entry was about me being busy around her apartment. I remember I was organizing her room and trying to make it homey. I should be glad she didn't write about her anger with me.

There are parts of me that wish she would've continued writing about her memory loss, if she were able. You never get to see her side of this disease. My most-treasured writing of hers was her last. She had a special note for me that I thought was going to be a loving note. As you remember, she said her nails looked bad. That was the end of her writing.

As you can imagine, her journals are special. Something that my girls will keep and will remind them of their grandma. They will note the entry of their births and how she talked about them with such love. I also can feel the love, reading about her own children and gratefulness for her life. I wish you could see all of them. She dearly loved her family, her hometown, her church, and her life as a mother, wife, sister, and friend.

Epilogue

The Healer, January 2016

Last month, I bought a Groupon for a massage/healer. It's the first Groupon I've ever purchased. I love to get a massage, yet I wasn't quite sure about the "healer" part of it. After I emailed back and forth with Kimberly, we set our appointment and I found out it was close to my work. There is nothing better than a massage.

I had a morning appointment and I was apprehensive because I wasn't sure where I was going. Her office is shared with another office (a therapist) and I wasn't sure if I was in the right place. I was starting to get nervous for some reason, worrying that I was the victim of a scam.

I arrived at the office and after waiting for about ten minutes, Kimberly came out and introduced herself. Her office was warm and inviting and smelled of lavender. I was nervous and did not know what to expect. But she put me at ease. She asked if I would lie on the table and I could stay fully dressed. I didn't need to get into a robe or crawl under the sheets?

She started to gently touch my feet and they suddenly became warm. Actually, I became warm all over. She was doing some reflexology on my feet and it felt good. If you have ever had your feet massaged, you know the feeling. In the meantime, she put something in my hands to hold, almost like a small upright weight. I'm sure she told me what it was, but I don't remember. Almost like a tuning fork?

I'm now wondering what kind of Groupon I have purchased, yet her rubbing my feet is pure heaven. Kimberly starts by saying, "When you walked in, so did a small, older woman with permed hair." She asked if my mom had died recently and I told her she has been gone since May of last year.

"You are not your mother's child." I'm confused. I said that I was my mother's child and then I remembered that I'm adopted. It's not something that I always carry with me or think about. She is quiet for a while and starts to talk about the cosmic world and energy.

"Did it take a long time for your parents to adopt you?" I answered that they tried for twenty years to have children but were not successful. She said that her being unsuccessful was meant to be and her adopting my brother and me was the cosmic universal plan. I was trying to take all of this in, trying to believe, but having a confusing conversation in my head. Do I believe this? She went on to say that it was meant to be that she brought me up and loved me in this world and that I helped her gracefully leave this world. She asked if I knew what this meant.

I did. Now she has my attention.

All this time she is gently touching my hip bones, my ear lobes, my forehead. I feel like my body is floating. I was trying to tell Steve that I was light as a feather. It was like whatever she was doing, my sadness and worry was leaving.

She also said that my mom likes to sit in Emme's chair at night. Now I'm a little scared. Emme's chair. For the past few months she has been having bad dreams. For a week straight, she woke up in the middle of the night. I'm not sure what is causing her distress. It's been hard for Emme, and I wasn't going to tell Kimberly anything, but I shared with her Emme's issue with her room.

She told me that my mom, Emme's grandma, watches out

for her and that she also loves my kitchen. I told her that made sense. My mom was a baker her whole life and loved our kitchen. Kimberly stated that I could talk to my mom and tell her to visit during the day and not the night, if it is scaring Emme. She feels that Emme is sensitive to things we cannot see. Super. That doesn't freak me out at all.

"Your mom also sends you love." And then I can feel the warm tears start to flow. She told me that she has crossed over and that she has a very important job. Her job is to take care of a big, beautiful garden and that she is the "greeter" for people who have crossed over. She waits in a tunnel and greets family and friends. Wow, that is a lot to take in.

She knew that my dad has been gone for a while and that his job was to help all of the veterans cross over. She also asked if our lights go on and off. That totally got me. I've shared with a few of you that our sunroom lights sporadically go on and off and that had never occurred before his death. Sometimes they will turn on, on command. This thoroughly freaks out only one person in our family. Me.

She laughed a little and said that my dad is a character (indeed) and that if it bothers me, he will stop. It was crazy that she knew that. I'm all right with it. If my family doesn't mind, I guess he can continue.

We talked about other things. She picked up that I help people cross over. I laughed a little because I hoped she didn't think that I really "cross" people over. She also laughed and said that she knew what I meant. She wanted to be sure that people didn't attach themselves to me after they have died. I'm freaked out again.

Finally, our visit of over an hour was done. I like to think of myself as very neutral thinking when it comes to healing, psychic things, and the unknown. I think all nurses have seen their fair share of strange, unexplainable things. Myself included. She lifted my soul a little, made me more peaceful. I kept thinking of our conversation. Sure, it's easy to read about someone. Maybe she read parts of my blog? But some things I do not talk about. She described my mom to a T and stated she is always around. That I could talk to her and she would hear me. That gave me peace.

My mom and I have talked since then. I asked her not to sit in Emme's chair at night but to still watch out for her. I told her it's all right to hang in our kitchen. I like that image. I told my dad that I will get used to his playfulness; my girls think it's funny.

In the end, I never got a "massage" but had a bit of healing that was unexpected. I never doubted that my parents would eventually be together again. I'm happy to know that they are enjoying being together. I truly believe that.

I hope they continue to look after our family and that they were proud of the things we did for them. Well, maybe except for the bathtub incident.

Acknowledgments

This book was written with so much love, and there are many people to thank for believing that I could actually write it.

Thank you to my family, Steve, Sophia, and Emme, for being a part of this journey, whether you wanted to or not. I'm so proud of you, Sophia and Emme, for loving your grandma the way you did and for giving her such joy and love all the way to the end. Steve, you didn't finish reading the whole book, but you had to live this with me every single day and I know it was just as hard for you as it was for me some days. Especially the bathroom part. I love you.

Thank you to Adam Wahlberg of Think Piece Publishing for believing in my story and for helping it along the way. You've helped me tremendously, just answering my annoying questions and encouraging me. I'm so glad Lisa Grantham introduced us. Much love and gratitude.

Thank you to my amazing editor, Anne Kelley Conklin, for all of your support and careful edits. We walked a very similar path in so many ways. Many, many thanks.

Thank you to my friends Dawn Barfnecht, Julie Hanson, and Leanne Peterson for being my first proofers. You ladies are so much smarter than I and took out parts that most likely made me sound crazy. I love that all three of you were so in sync. I'm so grateful for your help and friendship. Much love.

Thank you to my employer, and Tammy Sullivan, who had to put up with so much when I was taking care of my mom. Unexpected trips, emergency calls, tears shed, and worry while I was still trying to be a nurse. Thank you for all your advice and help while I was writing it. Bryan Sullivan, your "thank you" needs to come after Julie's. I love my job very much. Well, most days.

Thank you to my breakfast ladies, Leanne Peterson, Nichol Sutton, Dawn Barfnecht, Beth Mlekoday, Alana Erickson, and Jennefer Johnson, who have read just about as many books as I have. I adore all of you and you have been such a blessing to me. As friendships go, you are all the best. You've kept me together on more than one occasion.

Thank you to William Kent Krueger. While we were having coffee together, he asked me why I wanted to write this book. My answer is still the same, to help people. Even if it was just one person or family. You were, by far, my best auction purchase ever.

Much love to Wendy Doheny, who was one of the first believers in me. I could not ask for a better champion and sister. I love you.

Thank you to my brother, Ross Lundell.

Ryan Scheife, you are amazing in so many ways. Your wisdom, experience, patience, and professionalism is incredible. I appreciate everything you have done for me and helping to make the book what it is. I am deeply grateful. And that cover. Wow.

Melanie Liska, you helped me with the legal end of mom's issues more times than I can count. Thank you doesn't really sound like enough. Thank God you are the smarter one of us.

Everyone that was involved with taking care of Mom in memory care, thank you. Mickey, Amanda, Cathy, Kristi, Kelly, Patty, and so many wonderful nursing aides. Thank you to her assisted living staff, especially Carol and Grace. Heidi Brecht, thank you!

To the followers of my blog, The Lemon Bar Queen, thank you for lifting me up the days it was difficult. Your comments, suggestions, love, and encouragement were so important to me. I learned as much from you as you did from me. Trust me.

To all the families I have taken care of with any form of dementia. So many of you come to mind. I am so grateful you have allowed me to be your Nurse. On rare occasions I would share with you that my own mom had Alzheimer's disease. I could relate in so many ways and hopefully it helped you.

Thank you to the Alzheimer's Association for suggesting that I write my blog in the first place. This organization is near and dear to my heart. Our family has walked in their fundraiser more times than I can count. Research is important and so are funds. A portion of money from the sales of this book will go to The Alzheimer's Association. My mom would be happy to know that. Let's find a cure.

Thank you to my hometown of Starbuck, Minnesota, for looking after my mom for as long as you did. It sounds cliché to say it took a village, but it really did. There are too many people to thank but if you have a chance to visit midwestern Minnesota, please stop by the Dairy Queen in Starbuck and have a Blizzard or cone. It is truly the best Dairy Queen on the planet. Tell Carrie Brecht I sent you.

Lastly, somewhere high above, I hope my parents are happy with the story I've told and are proud of me. I miss their love. Thank you for all you have done for me. I'm so grateful you picked me as your daughter.

Favorite Recipes

by Jeanne Lundell

Lemon Bars

- ❏ 2 cups flour
- ❏ 1 cup butter or margarine
- ❏ ½ cup powdered sugar

Mix together and press into bottom of 8x8-inch pan.
Bake 30 minutes at 325°F.

Beat 4 eggs and add 2 cups of sugar. Then add:

- ❏ 4 Tbsp. flour
- ❏ 4 Tbsp. lemon juice
- ❏ 1 tsp. baking powder

Pour onto the baked crust and bake for 30 minutes more.

Rhubarb Dessert (Jodi's favorite!)

Crust:

- ❑ 1 cup flour
- ❑ 2 Tbsp. sugar
- ❑ ½ cup butter
- ❑ ¼ cup chopped nuts (optional)

Mix and press into 8x8-inch pan. Bake 15–20 minutes at 325°F.

Filling:

- ❑ 2 ½ cups rhubarb, cut up
- ❑ 3 egg yolks and reserve 3 egg whites
- ❑ 1 cup sugar
- ❑ ⅓ cup cream or evaporated milk
- ❑ 2 Tbsp. flour

Pour over crust and bake 40 minutes at 325°.
Beat 3 egg whites. Add 6 Tbsp. sugar.
Pour over baked rhubarb mixture and bake until brown.

Buttermilk Potato Doughnuts

- ❑ 1 ½ cups hot unseasoned mashed potatoes
- ❑ ½ cup melted butter or margarine
- ❑ 2 cups sugar
- ❑ 3 eggs
- ❑ 1 cup buttermilk
- ❑ 1 tsp. vanilla
- ❑ 5 ½ cups flour
- ❑ 4 tsp. baking powder
- ❑ 1 ½ tsp. baking soda
- ❑ 1 tsp. salt
- ❑ 1 tsp. ground nutmeg
- ❑ 2 cups sugar

Combine potatoes, butter, sugar, eggs, buttermilk, and vanilla. Beat until well blended. Sift together flour, baking powder, baking soda, salt, and nutmeg. Gradually stir dry ingredients into potato mixture, blending well after each addition. Chill for one hour. Drop rounded teaspoonfuls of dough into hot oil (360ºF). Brown on one side, turn, and brown on the other. Drain on paper towels. Roll in sugar. Makes six dozen.

Pumpkin Torte

Crust:

- ❑ 24 graham crackers, crushed
- ❑ ½ cup butter
- ❑ ⅓ cup sugar

Mix crackers, butter, and sugar and press into 9x13-inch pan.

Filling:

- ❑ 2 eggs
- ❑ 8 oz. cream cheese, softened
- ❑ ¾ cup sugar

Mix and pour over crust. Bake 20 minutes at 350°F.

Layer 2:

- ❑ 2 cups pumpkin
- ❑ 3 egg yolks and reserve the 3 egg whites
- ❑ ½ cup sugar
- ❑ ½ cup milk
- ❑ ½ tsp. salt
- ❑ 1 Tbsp. cinnamon
- ❑ 1 envelope plain gelatin
- ❑ ¼ cup cold water
- ❑ ¼ cup sugar
- ❑ ½ pint whipping cream

Cook pumpkin, egg yolks, ½ cup sugar, milk, salt, and cinnamon until mixture thickens. Remove from heat and add gelatin dissolved in ¼ cup cold water. Cool. Beat egg whites and ¼ cup sugar and fold into pumpkin mixture. Pour over cooled baked crust. Top with whipped cream.

Rhubarb Cream Pie

- ❏ 1 ½ cups sugar
- ❏ 3 Tbsp. flour
- ❏ ½ tsp. nutmeg
- ❏ 1 Tbsp. butter
- ❏ 2 beaten eggs
- ❏ 3 cups rhubarb, cut up
- ❏ Pie pastry, top and bottom

Combine sugar, flour, nutmeg, and butter. Add eggs and beat until smooth. Add rhubarb. Pour into 9-inch pastry-lined pie pan. Top with pastry. Bake in hot oven (450°F) for 10 minutes, then in moderate oven (350°F) for 30 minutes.